Disclaimer: This textbook is not intended to provide, and disclaims any suggestion that it does provide, medical advice of any nature. The information made available through this textbook should not be used in place of seeking professional opinions by licensed practitioners. Only licensed medical professionals may offer medical advice, diagnosis and recommendations for treatment of medical conditions. You assume full responsibility for appropriate use of the information available through this textbook.

As Medicine is an ever-changing science, with new research and clinical experience, changes in treatment and techniques are required. The author(s) has (have) checked with sources believed to be reliable in effort to provide information that is complete and generally in accord with standards accepted at the time of publication. The opinions expressed in this work represent those of the author(s) and, in view of the possibility of human error or changes in medical science, neither the author(s), RAEducation.com LLC, nor any other party who has been involved in the preparation or publication of this work warrants that the information contained herein is in every respect accurate or complete and they are not responsible for any errors or omissions or for the results obtained from the use of such information. Readers and viewers are encouraged to confirm the information contained herein with other sources.

Published by RAEducation.com LLC Publications, Gainesville, FL USA
Produced by Kristine Lyle, Printers Workshop, Kalona, IA

ISBN-10:   1-948083-00-0
ISBN-13:   978-1-948083-00-3

André P. Boezaart

MBChB, MPraxMed, DA(CMSA), FFA(CMSA), MMed(Anesth), PhD
Professor of Anesthesiology and Orthopaedic Surgery
Chief of Division of Acute and Peri-operative Pain Medicine
Chief of Acute Pain Service
University of Florida College of Medicine, Gainesville, Florida, USA

Co-Author:

Donald S. Bohannon, MD

Associate Professor of Anesthesiology
Dept of Anesthesiology
Division of Acute and Perioperative Pain Medicine
University of Florida College of Medicine, Gainesville, FL, USA

Artwork by:
Mary K. Bryson, MAMS, CMI
Bryson Biomedical Illustration
Langhorne, Pennsylvania

Educational electronic and printed media for the website
RAEducation.com owned by RAEducation.com LLC.

Please visit www.RAEducation.com
for video tutorials on this and other topics

The Cervical Paravertebral Block

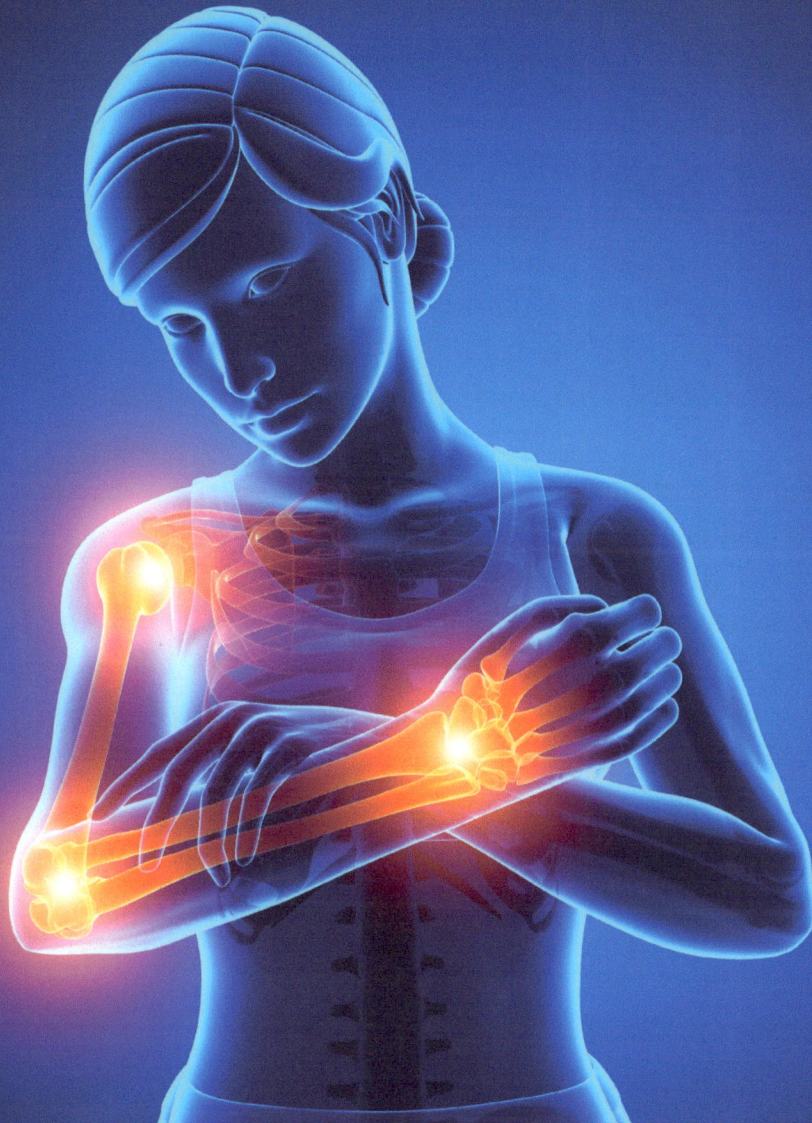

Preface

Welcome to this series on High-yield Nerve Blocks. These are nerve blocks that are essential blocks required as a minimum for the practice of modern Acute and Perioperative Pain Medicine. A high-yield block is one that, when properly performed, poses minimum risks versus maximum benefits, in other words they are blocks that give you (and more important, the patient) maximum bang for your buck. There are essentially only a handful of such blocks, and if they are completely mastered, a practitioner can manage the acute pain and perioperative pain associate with most, if not all, clinical situations. The other blocks are described on the RAEducation.com website if you need to do one for some clinical reason.

The high-yield blocks are extensively covered in this series in great detail; each block starting with a PART 1 that deals with Applied Anatomy and followed by the Technique itself in detail as a PART 2. It has to be emphasized that in depth anatomical knowledge is key and central to successful Acute Pain Medicine and Regional Anesthesia. If a practitioner truly understands the Applied Anatomy, they do not really have to study the technique, because they already know how to do the block. Study the technique anyway, because this series will provide you with small (or large) nuances of the block to make you even more successful.

All the blocks and macro-, micro-, sono-, and functional anatomy and pharmacology referred to in this series are discussed in much more detail on the RAEducation.com website (www. RAEducation.com). There are complete instructional videos on exactly how to perform all the high-yield (and other) blocks as well as video tutorials on detailed anatomy, pharmacology, and a host of other topics.

André P. Boezaart

Part 1: Applied Anatomy

Essentially, as for all 4 paravertebral blocks; the cervical (CPVB), the thoracic (TPVB), the lumbar (LPVB)and the sacral paravertebral block (SPVB) (Fig. 1a-d), the technique is principally the same and based on the same anatomical principles.

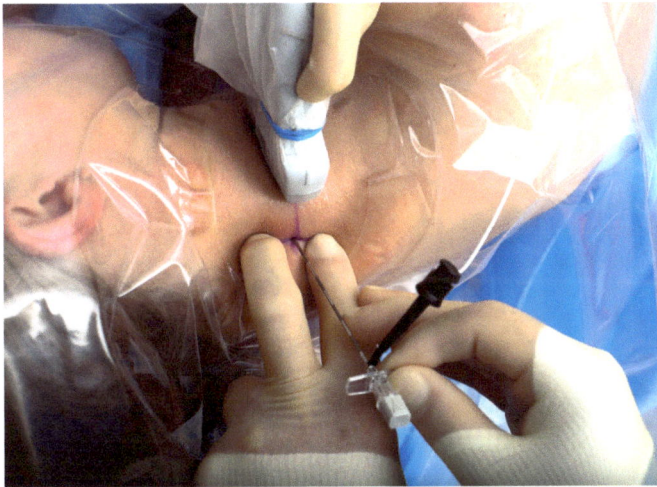

Figure 1a: Cervical Paravertebral Block

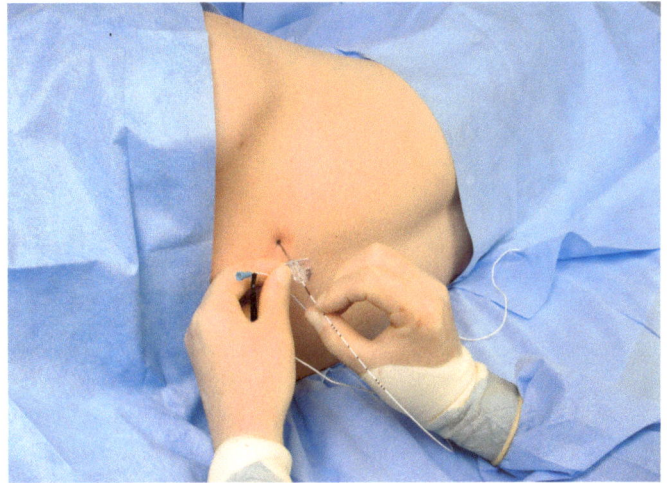

Figure 1b: Thoracic Paravertebral Block

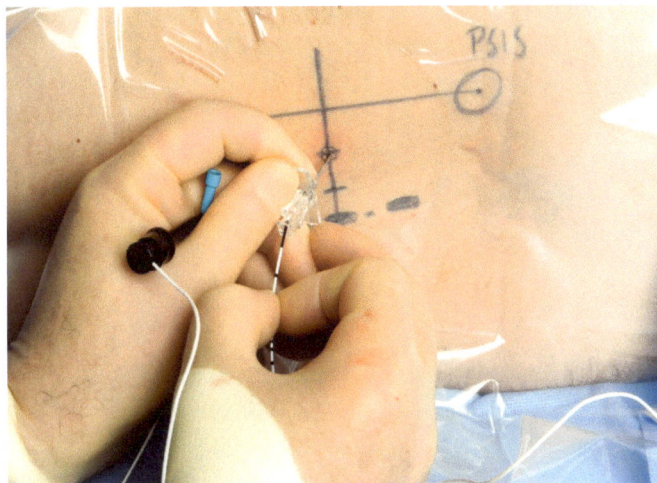

Figure 1c: Lumbar Paravertebral Block

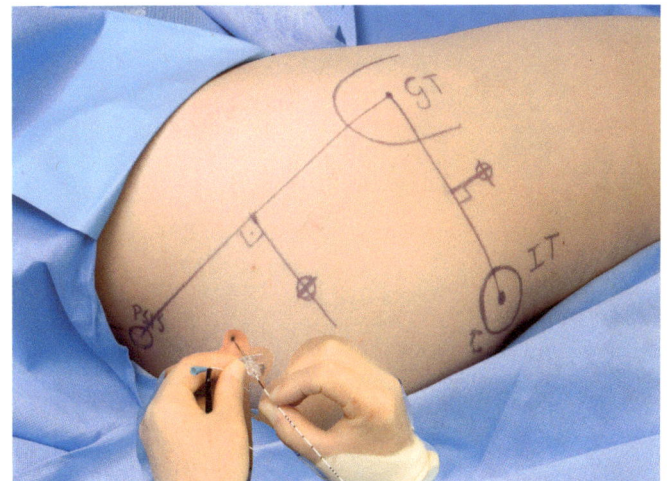

Figure 1d: Sacral Paravertebral Block

All the paravertebral blocks are based on 6 anatomical steps:

1.   After anatomically identifying the external landmarks with or without ultrasound, we place the needle tip against some bony landmark. This gives the operator a bony landmark and indication of depth from which to proceed with confidence. In the case of the cervical paravertebral block, this is the posterior tubercle of the transverse process of C7 (Fig. 2a & b). For the TPVB (Fig. 2c) and LPVB (Fig. 2d) this is the transverse process of the appropriate vertebra, and for the SPVB (Fig 2e) it is the ala or wing of the ilium or sacrum.

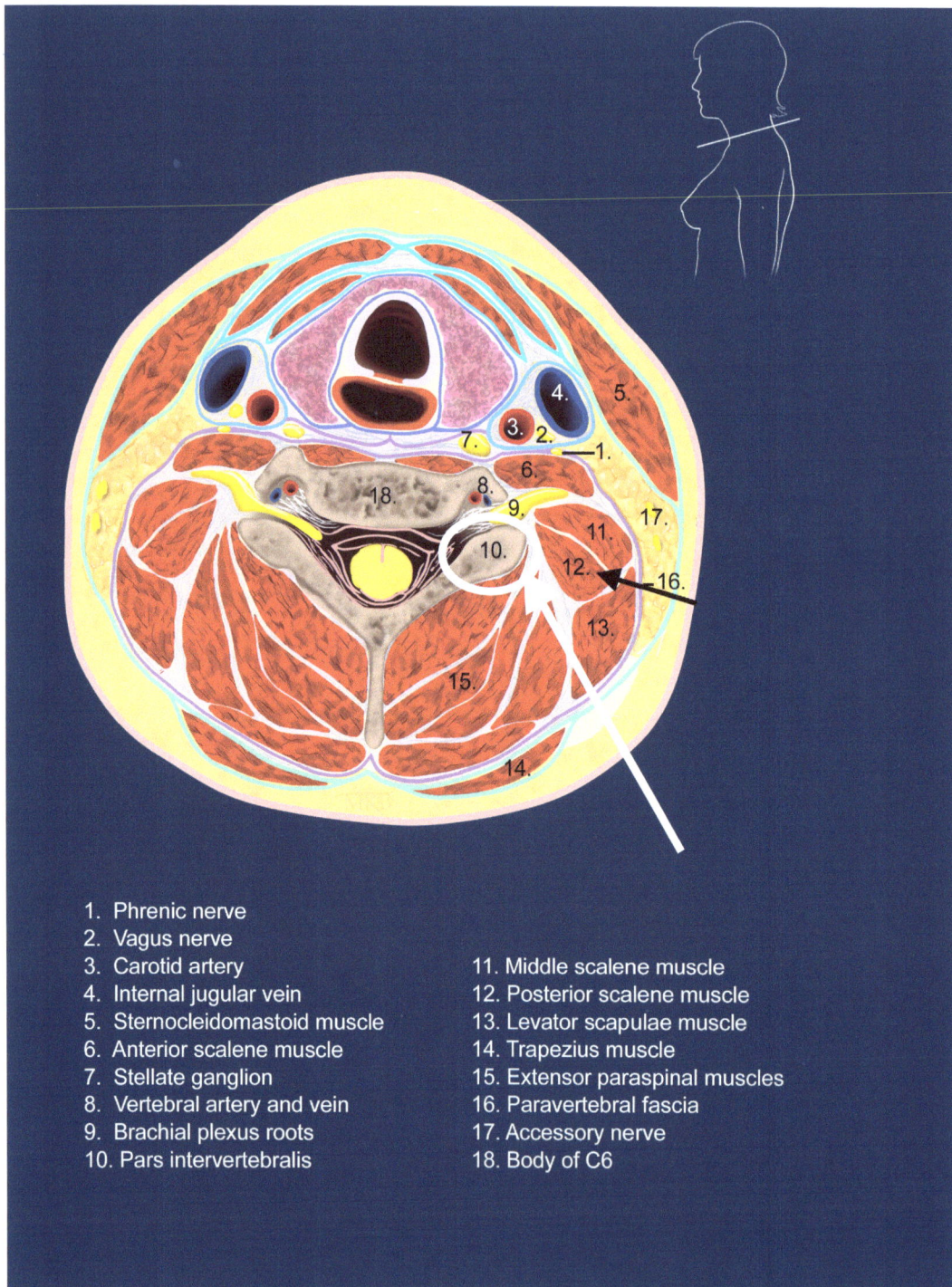

1. Phrenic nerve
2. Vagus nerve
3. Carotid artery
4. Internal jugular vein
5. Sternocleidomastoid muscle
6. Anterior scalene muscle
7. Stellate ganglion
8. Vertebral artery and vein
9. Brachial plexus roots
10. Pars intervertebralis
11. Middle scalene muscle
12. Posterior scalene muscle
13. Levator scapulae muscle
14. Trapezius muscle
15. Extensor paraspinal muscles
16. Paravertebral fascia
17. Accessory nerve
18. Body of C6

Figure 2a:

Reprinted with permission from Andre P Boezaart Primer of Regional Anesthesia Anatomy, 2nd Ed, and Mary K Bryson

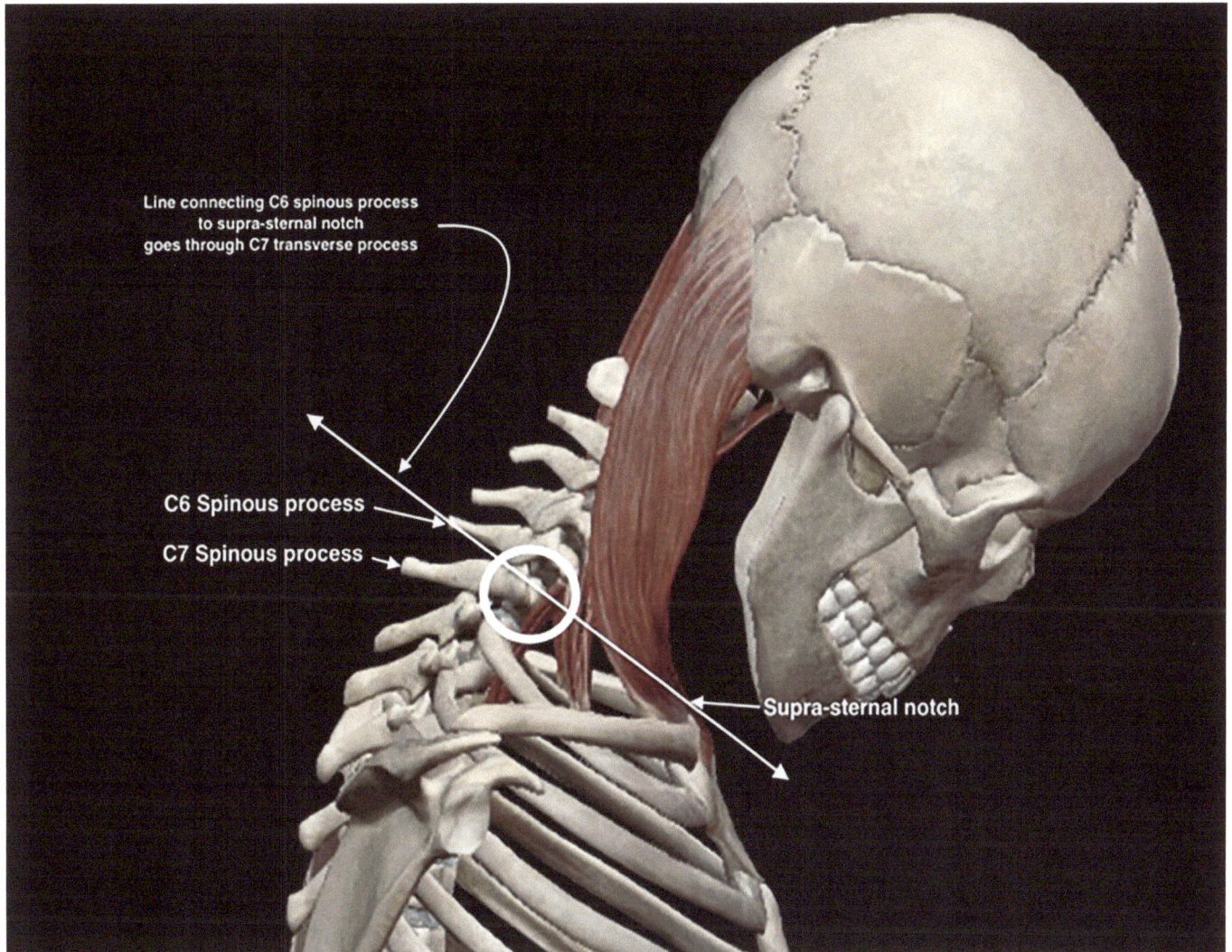

Line connecting C6 spinous process to supra-sternal notch goes through C7 transverse process

C6 Spinous process

C7 Spinous process

Supra-sternal notch

Figure 2b

For the CPVB, the needle (white arrow in Fig 2a) walks off laterally of the posterior tubercle of the transverse process of C7 (white oval, #10 on Fig. 2a) and enters the tendinous fibers of the posterior scalene muscle (black arrow, #12 on Fig. 2a)

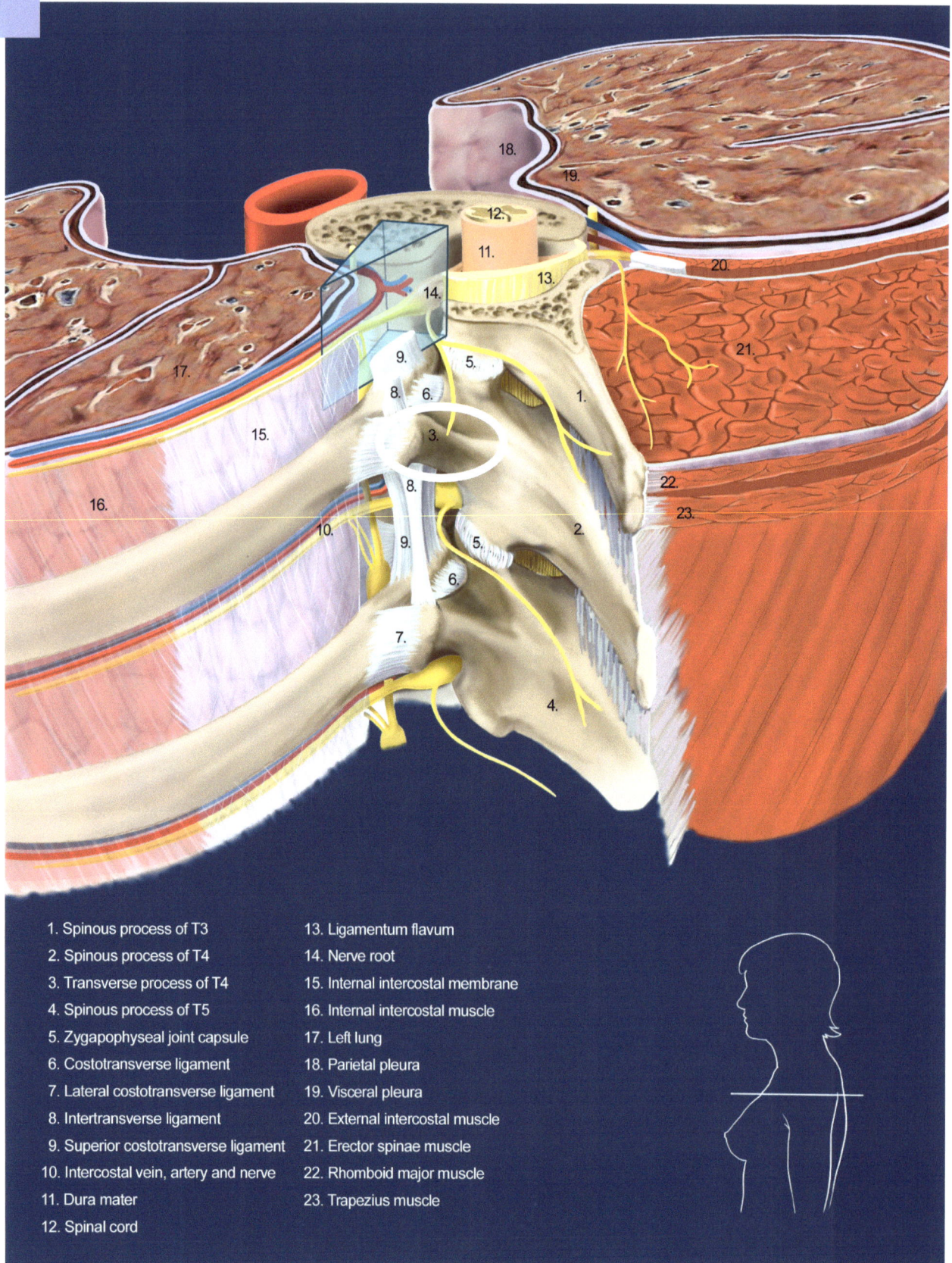

1. Spinous process of T3
2. Spinous process of T4
3. Transverse process of T4
4. Spinous process of T5
5. Zygapophyseal joint capsule
6. Costotransverse ligament
7. Lateral costotransverse ligament
8. Intertransverse ligament
9. Superior costotransverse ligament
10. Intercostal vein, artery and nerve
11. Dura mater
12. Spinal cord

13. Ligamentum flavum
14. Nerve root
15. Internal intercostal membrane
16. Internal intercostal muscle
17. Left lung
18. Parietal pleura
19. Visceral pleura
20. External intercostal muscle
21. Erector spinae muscle
22. Rhomboid major muscle
23. Trapezius muscle

Fig 2c

For the TPVB, the needle walks off the transverse process (white oval) of the vertebra and enters the costotransverse ligament.

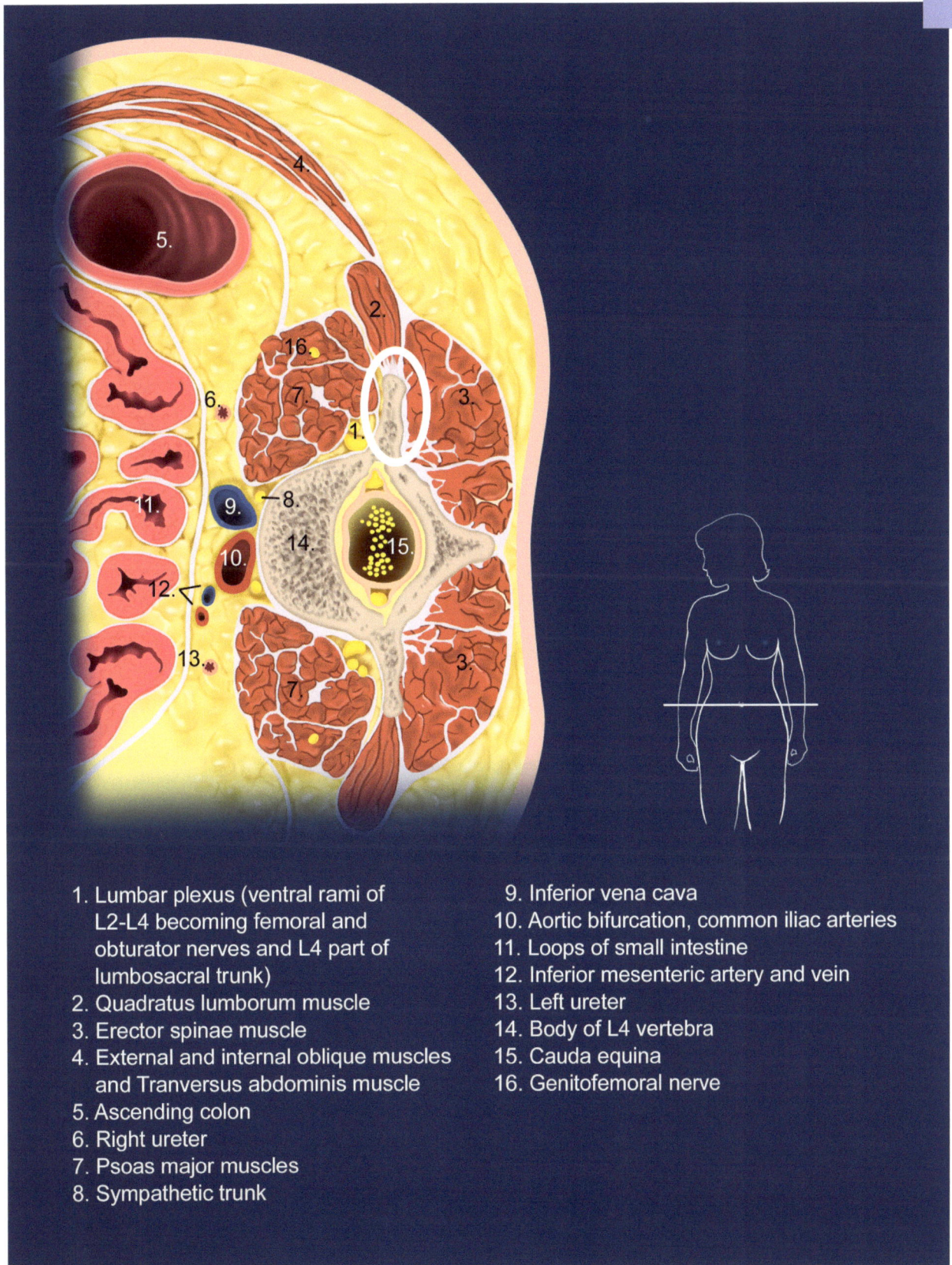

Fig 2d

1. Lumbar plexus (ventral rami of L2-L4 becoming femoral and obturator nerves and L4 part of lumbosacral trunk)
2. Quadratus lumborum muscle
3. Erector spinae muscle
4. External and internal oblique muscles and Tranversus abdominis muscle
5. Ascending colon
6. Right ureter
7. Psoas major muscles
8. Sympathetic trunk
9. Inferior vena cava
10. Aortic bifurcation, common iliac arteries
11. Loops of small intestine
12. Inferior mesenteric artery and vein
13. Left ureter
14. Body of L4 vertebra
15. Cauda equina
16. Genitofemoral nerve

For the LPVB, the needle walks off the transverse process of the vertebra (white oval) and enters the anterior fascia of the quadratus lumborum muscle.

Reprinted with permission from Andre P Boezaart Primer of Regional Anesthesia Anatomy, 2nd Ed, and Mary K Bryson

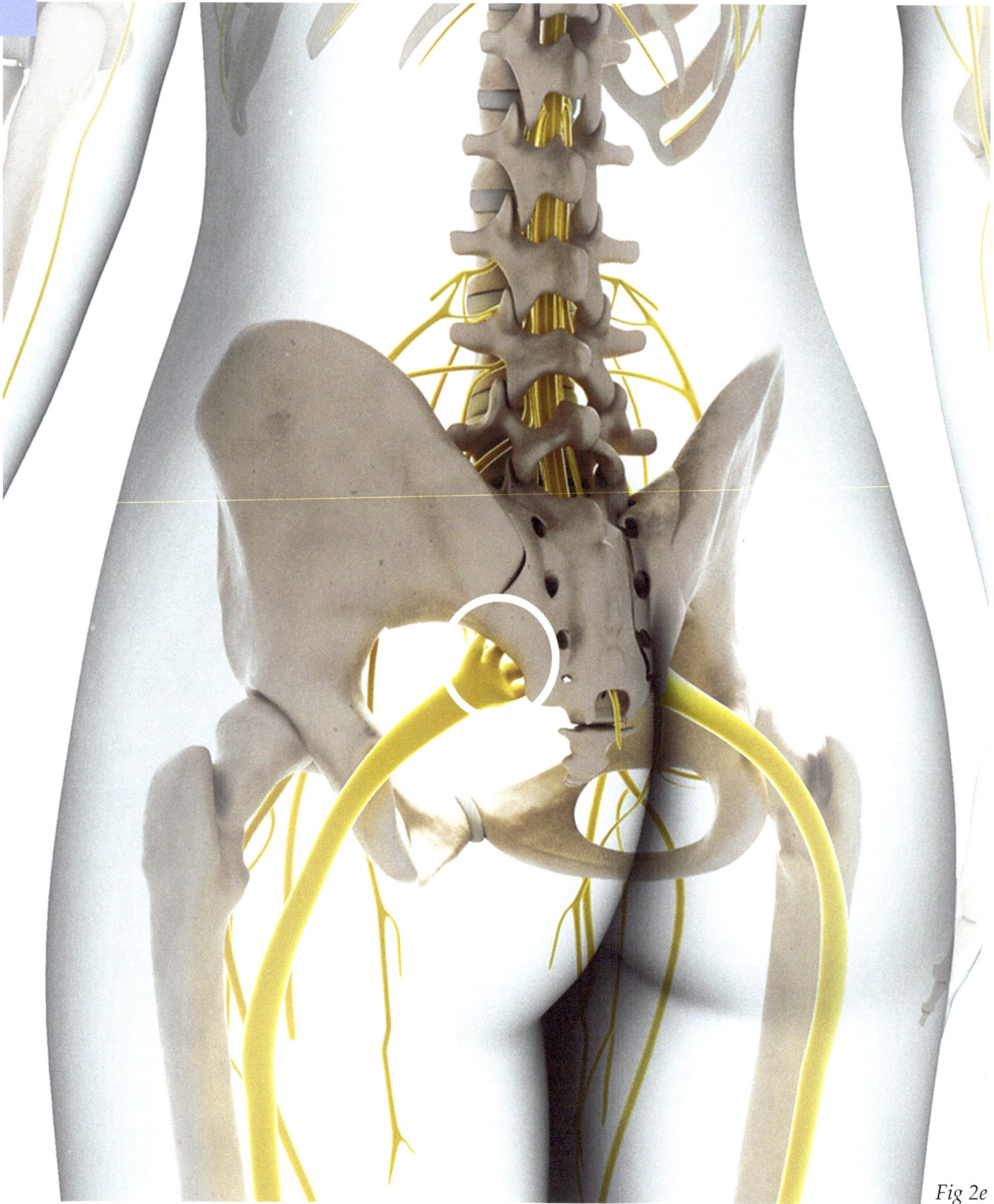

Fig 2e

For the SPVB, the needle walks off the sacrum or ala of the ilium and enters the greater sciatic notch.

2. The needle tip is then "walked off" this bony structure or landmark (laterally, in the case of the cervical paravertebral block) and…

3. Advanced anteriorly through a dense tissue with a high resistance to air or 5% dextrose in water (D5W) – the slips of origin of the posterior scalene muscle, which are tendinous in the case of the CPVB. (See page 10-11, Figs 2a-b) For the TPVB, this dense tissue is the costo-transverse ligament, (See page 12, Fig 2c) and for the LPVB the anterior fascia of the quadratus lumborum muscle. (Seepage 13, Fig 2d)

4. Loss of resistance (to air or D5W) is encountered as the needle exits anterior to this dense tissue.

5. The needle is then advanced anteriorly approximately one-half to 1 cm to encounter the C6 root (biceps motor response) for shoulder surgery, or slightly more caudal to the C7 root (triceps motor response) for elbow and wrist surgery. It encounters the thoracic spinal roots, lumbar plexus and sacral plexus respectively for the TPVB, LPVB and SPVB.

6. And finally, a catheter for a continuous nerve block is placed in the "sweet spot" of the nerve, believed to be inside the sub-circumneural space – also known as the sub-paraneural space in older texts.

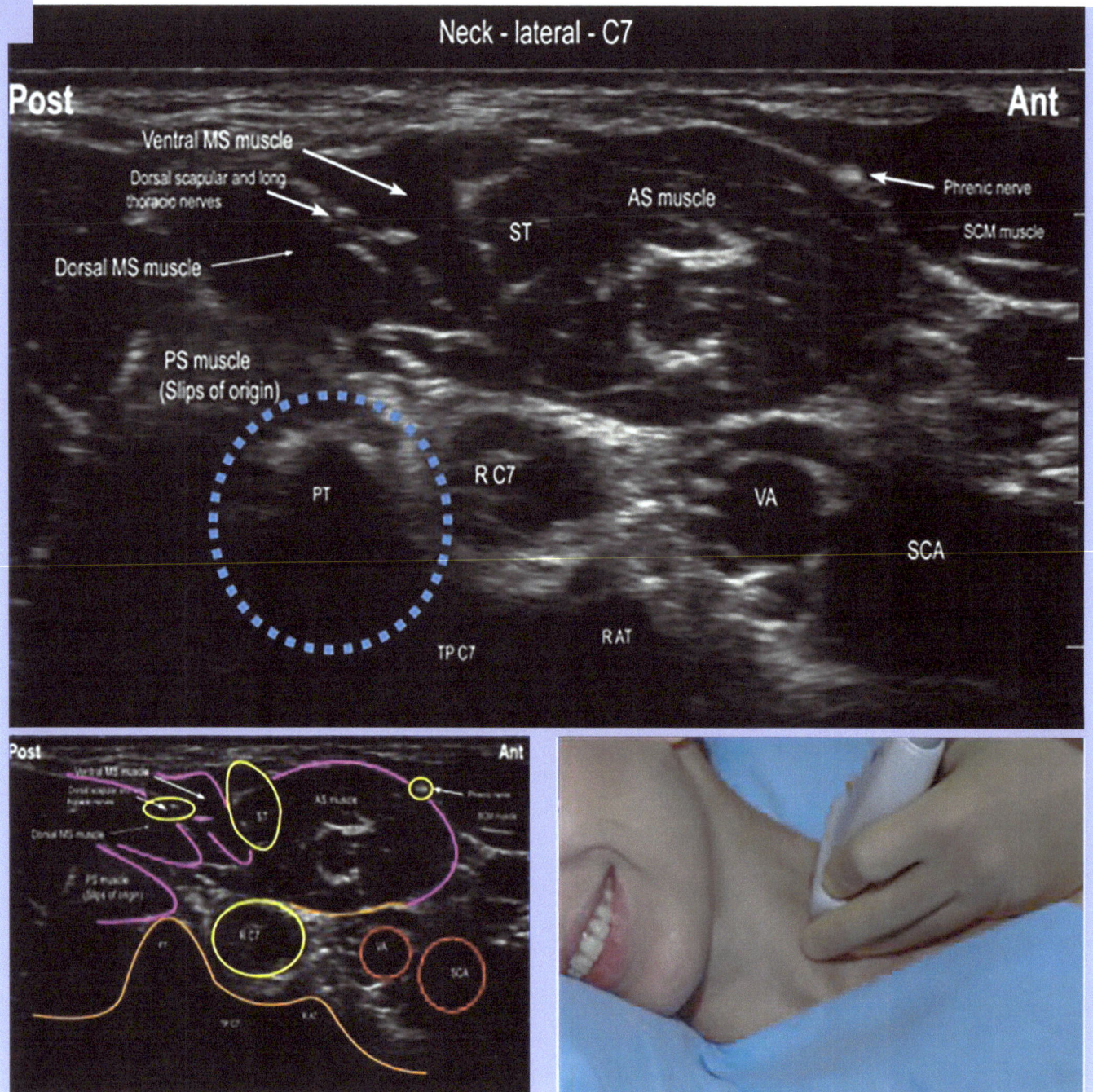

Figure 3: Sonogram of the lateral aspect of the neck at the level of C7. The light blue circle (PT) indicates the posterior tubercle of the transverse process of C7, while RAT indicates the rudimentary anterior process.

Unlike the other cervical vertebrae, the transverse process of the 7th cervical vertebra does not have an anterior tubercle (or it is rudimentary), which makes it distinct and easy to identify with ultrasound.

AS	Anterior scalene muscle
MS	Middle scalene muscle
PS	Posterior scalene muscle
PT	posterior tubercle of the transverse process of C7
RAT	rudimentary anterior process
RC7	spinal root of C7
SCA	Subclavian Artery
SCM	Sternocleidomastoid muscle
ST	Superior trunk
TPC7	Transverse process of C7
VA	Vertebral Artery

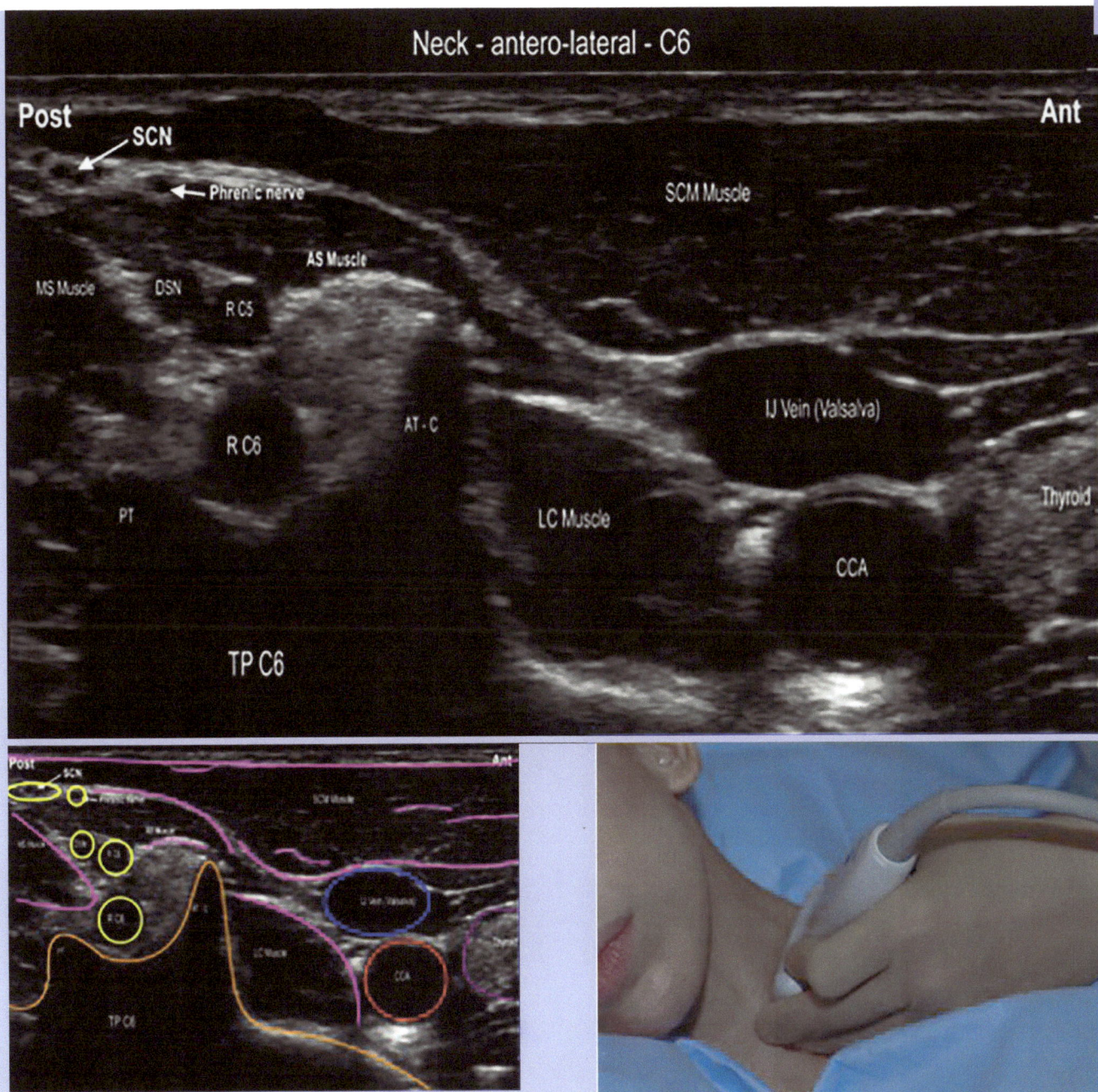

Figure 4: Sonogram of the lateral aspect of the neck at the level of C6. AT-C indicates prominent anterior (or Carotid, or Chassaignac's) tubercle

The C6 transverse process, on the other hand, usually has a large anterior tubercle sometimes called the carotid tubercle or Chassaignac's tubercle.

AS	Anterior scalene muscle
AT-C	Anterior Carotid (Chassaignac's) tubercle
CCA	Common carotid artery
LCMuscle	Longus colli muscle
MS	Middle scalene muscle
DSN	Dorsal scapular nerve
IJ	Internal jugular
PT	Posterior tubercle
RC5	spinal root of C5
RC6	spinal root of C6
SCM	Sternocleidomastoid muscle
SCN	Supraclavicular nerves
TPC6	Transverse process of C6

Surface Anatomy and Landmarks

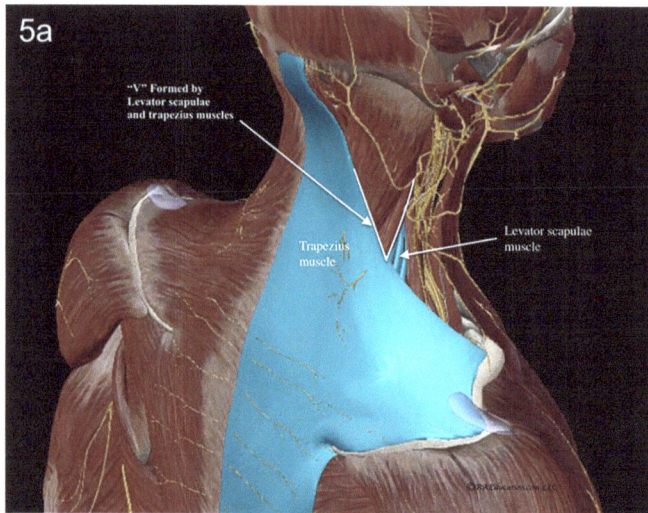

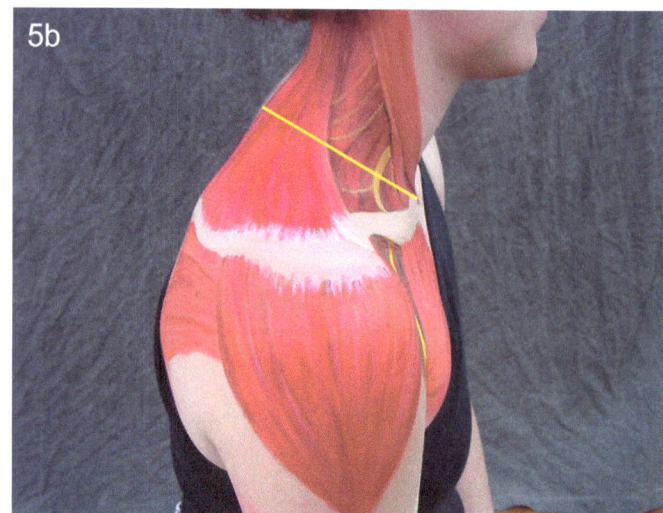

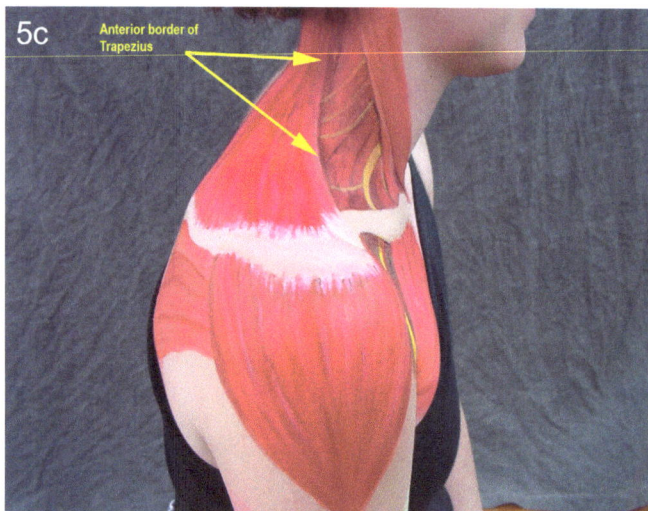

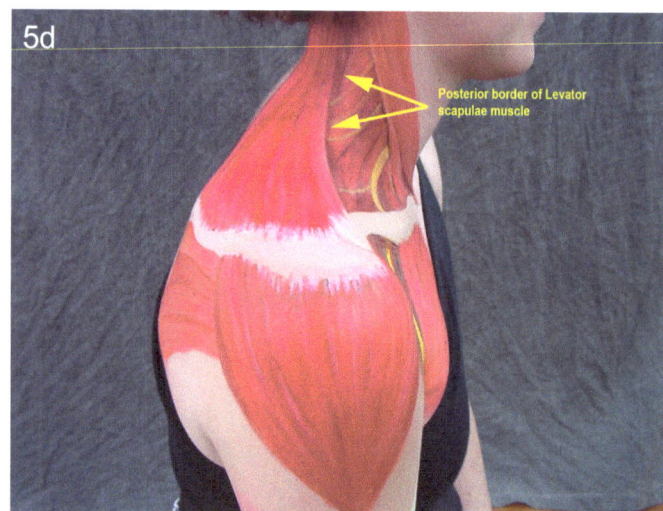

Figure 5a, b, c & d: There is a "V" forming a groove between the trapezius and levator scapulae muscles

There are two ways to get to the posterior tubercle of the transverse process of C7:

1.   With anatomical landmarks
2.   With ultrasound assistance

For the anatomical landmark method, which I would encourage readers to use even if they use ultrasound to find the bony landmark, we follow the groove behind the mastoid process caudad. There is a "V" formed by the anterior border of the trapezius muscle and the posterior border of the levator scapulae muscle

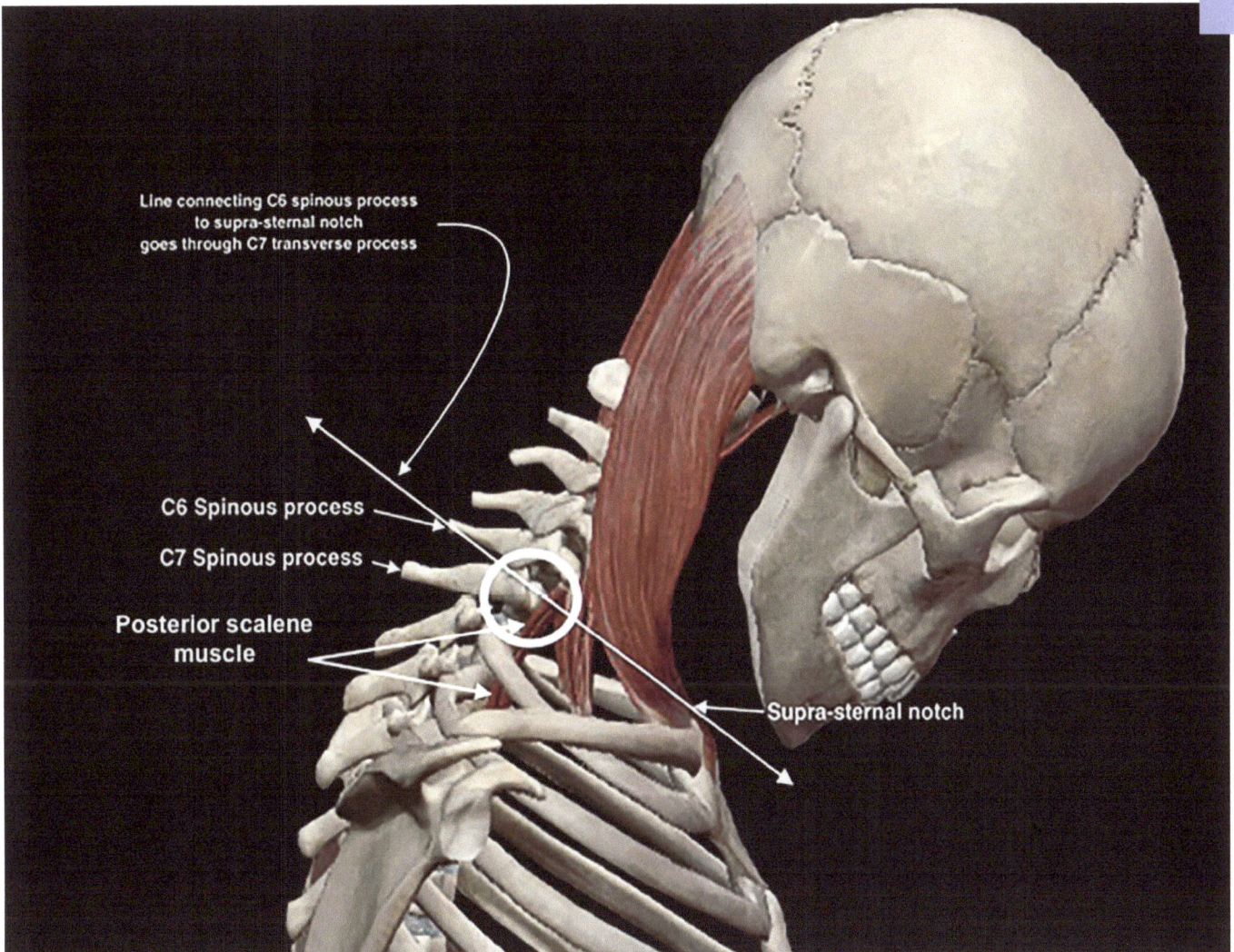

Figure 6a: A line drawn from the spinous process of C6 to the suprasternal notch goes through the posterior. tubercle of the transverse process of C7 (White Circle).

We can identify the C6 spinous process - the one above the prominent C7 - and draw a line from it to the suprasternal notch. With the head flexed anteriorly, this line, when viewed from the lateral, goes through the posterior tubercle of the transverse process of the 7th cervical vertebra (White Circle Shown in Fig. 6a). If the probe of an ultrasound is placed on this line (Fig. 6b), the PTTP C7 comes into view (Fig. 6c).

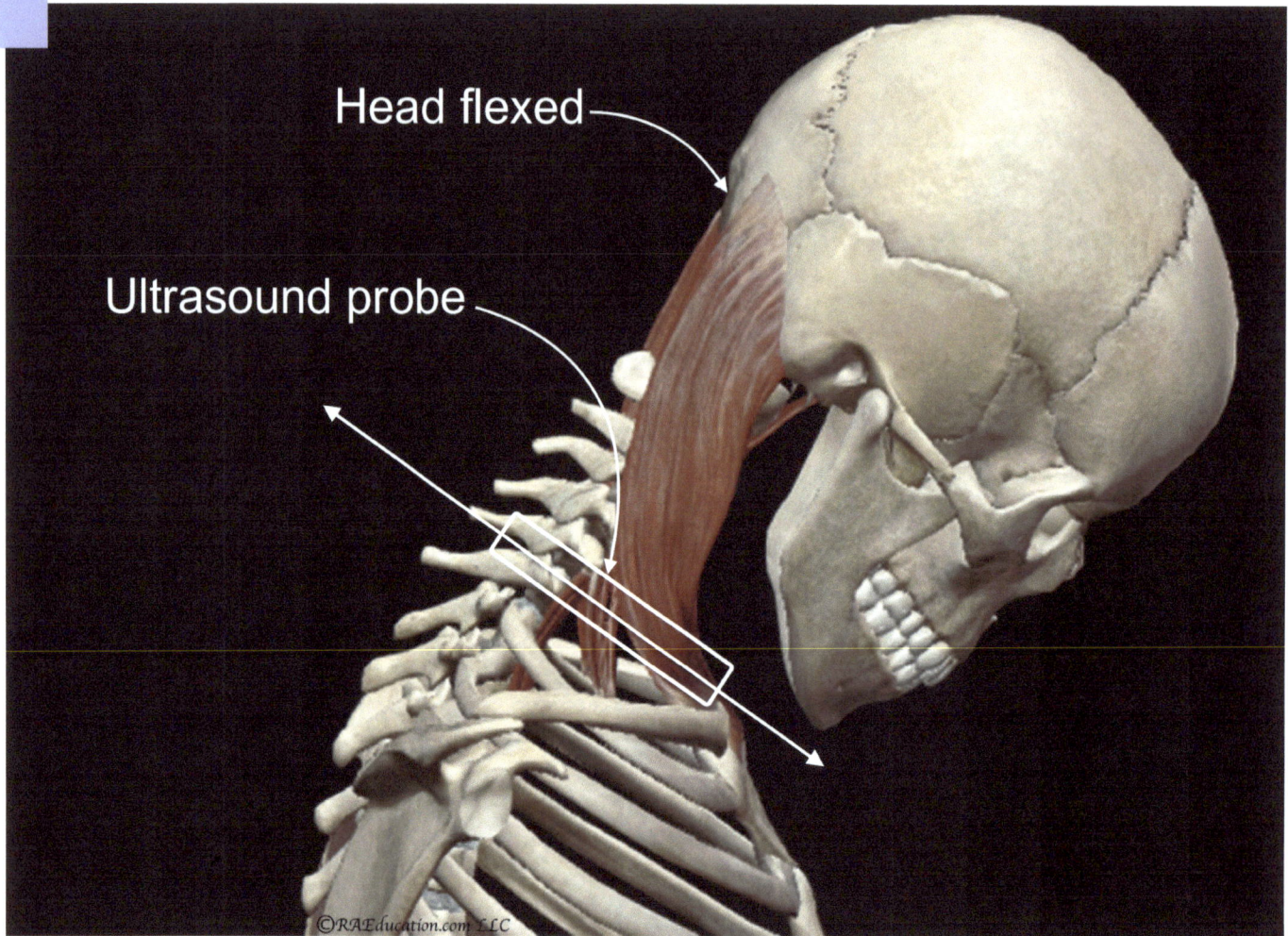

Head flexed

Ultrasound probe

©RAEducation.com LLC

Figure 6b: Ultrasound probe placed on line joining C6 spinous process with suprasternal notch.

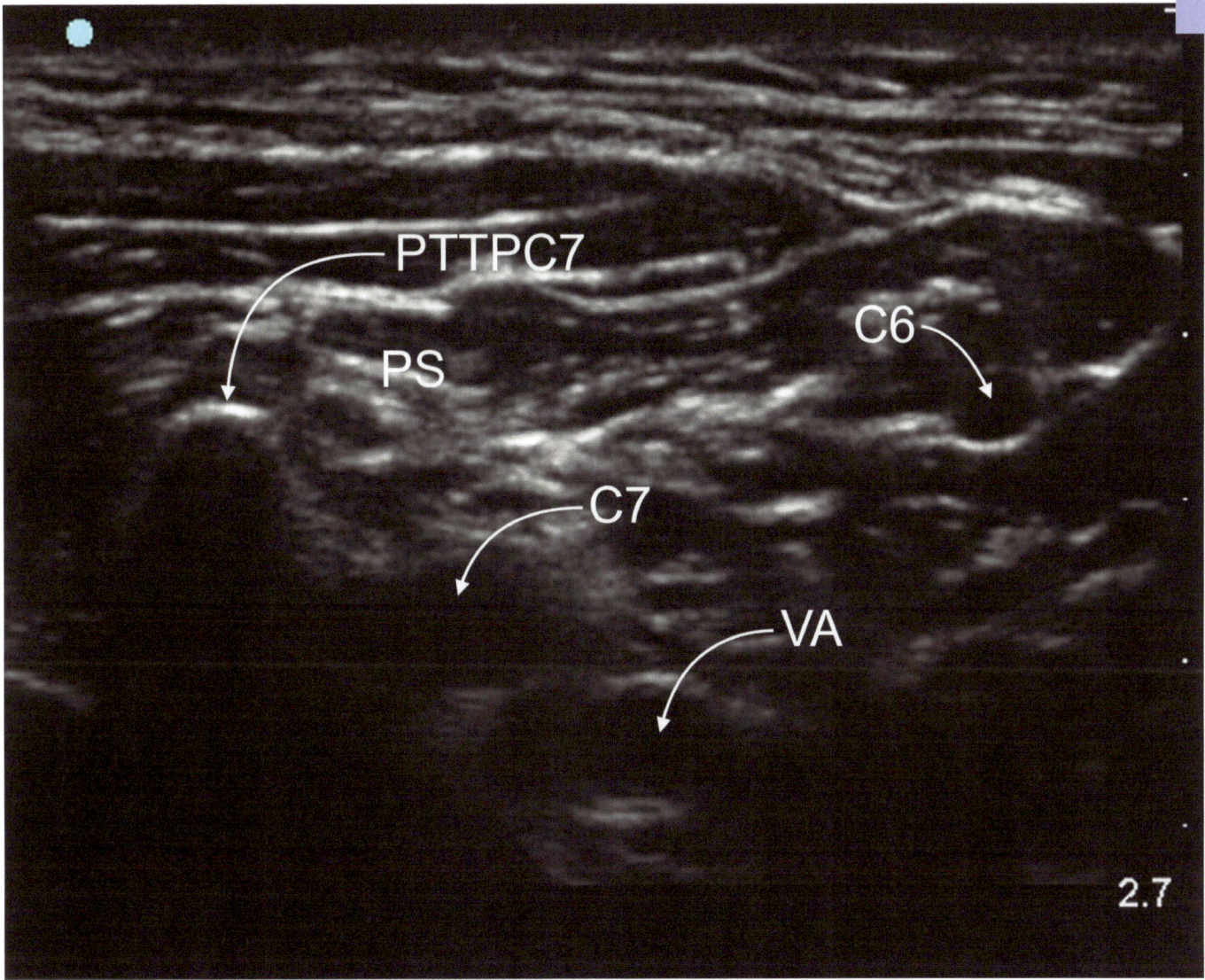

Figure 6c:

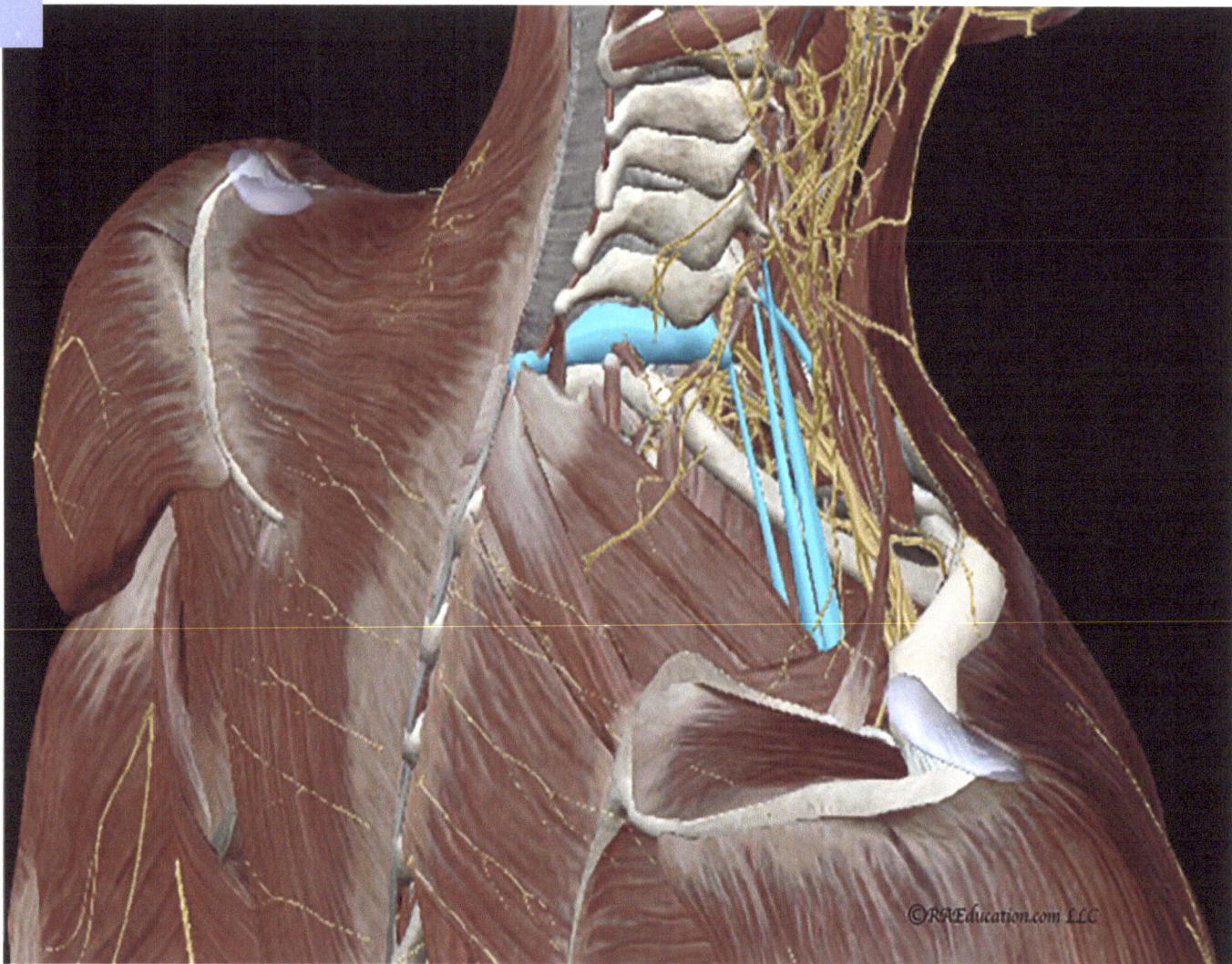

©RAEducation.com LLC

Figure 7: The slips of origin on the posterior scalene muscles are tendonous at this level and are indicated here in light blue. The 7th cervical vertebra is also colored light blue. The posterior scalene muscle implants proximally on the posterior tubercles of the C5, C6 and C7 transverse processes and distally on the 2nd rib.

"Walk off" laterally of this bony landmark, the posterior tubercle of the transverse process of C7, and the needle tip enters the tendinous or aponeurotic dense part of the slips of origin of the posterior scalene muscle, marked in light blue, which implant on the posterior tubercles of the transverse processes of C5, C6, and C7 proximally and the 2nd rib distally.

As the needle is advanced anteriorly, the needle tip exits anterior to the posterior scalene muscle and we encounter a distinct loss of resistance to air or 5% dextrose in water. If we use saline, the nerve stimulator will not evoke a motor response anymore. The C6 spinal root will be encountered after advancing the needle tip a few more millimeters, but seldom more than one centimeter (Figs. 8 & 6c).

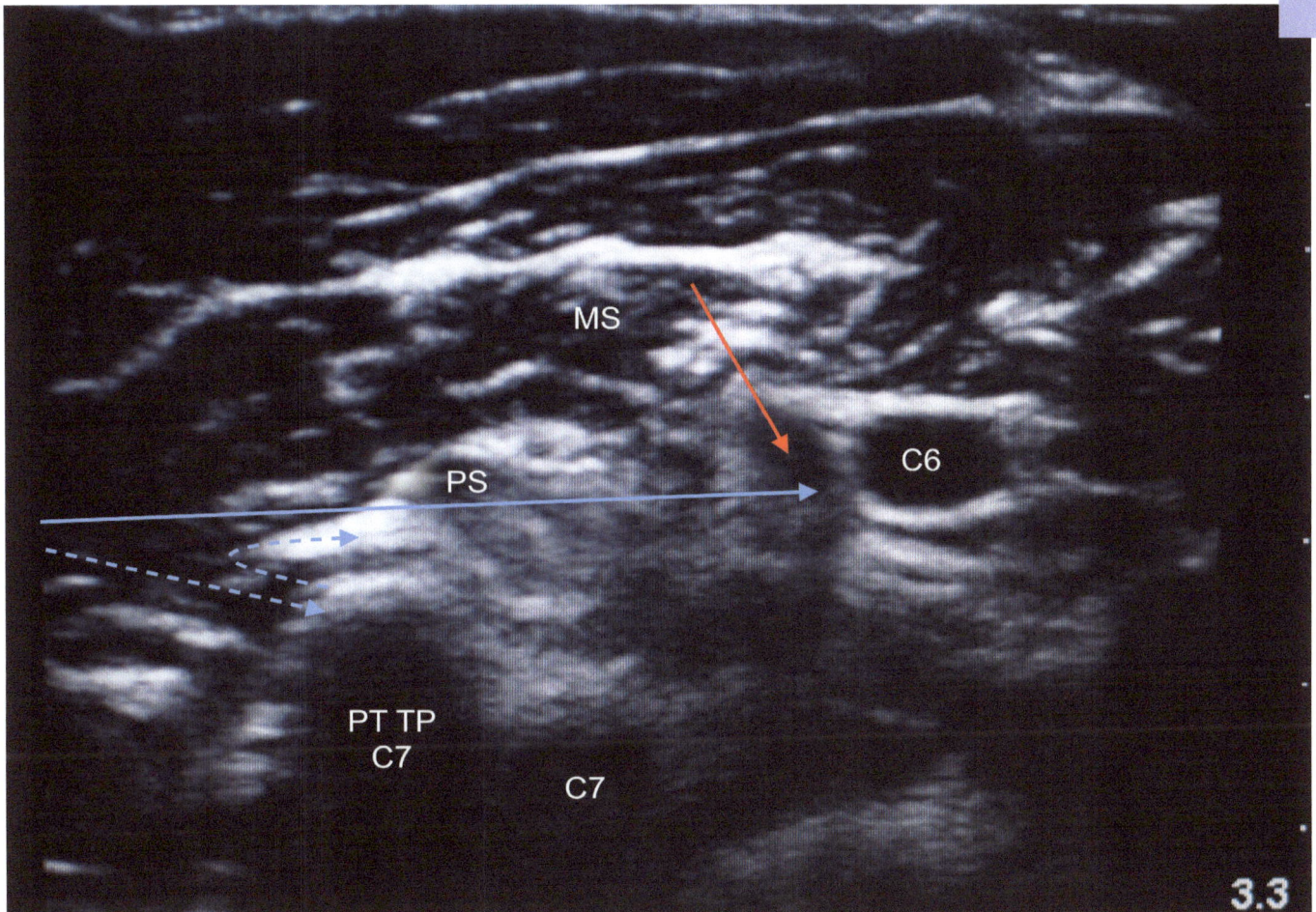

Figure 8: A sonogram of the lateral part of the lower neck with the ultrasound probe placed on the line joining the C6 spinous process and the suprasternal notch.

Please note the position of the slips of origin of the posterior scalene muscle (PS). See that it is much denser (more white or echogenic) than middle scalene muscle (MS), which is more "fleshy" (less tendinous) at this level.

The needle (light blue arrow) walks off laterally of the posterior tubercle and advances through the dense posterior scalene muscle, where there is resistance to air, until it reaches the anterior border of the posterior scalene muscle and exits the muscle where a distinct loss of resistance is encountered at the red arrow. This is immediately followed by a biceps muscle motor response as the C6 root is electrically stimulated.

(If the surgery is more distal – elbow or wrist, the needle entry is more caudad and the C7 spinal root is targeted and a triceps motor response is sought).

C6	C6 spinal root
C7	C7 spinal root
MS	Middle scalene muscle (dorsal head)
PS	Posterior scalene muscle (slips of origin)
PTTPC7	Posterior tubercle of the transverse process of the 7th cervical vertebra
- - - ▶	initial trajectory of Tuohy needle after encountering the PTTPC7
▬▬▶	final trajectory of Tuohy needle
▬▬▶	Exit of posterior scalene muscle where loss of resistance is encountered.
3.3	depth in cm

increasing number of authors have noted the relevance of counterfactual models to ecological studies of the effect of potentially mutable factors on disease occurrence.

To obtain more than fragmentary knowledge of causes and their effects (for example, the causes of obesity at the molecular, cellular, individual, neighborhood, or societal levels), a causal model or theoretical framework is needed. Ecological models of disease causation are an important example of this. As Cartwright [2] noted, although much of our warranted causal information comes in bits and pieces, what is needed for policy is the whole picture.

HOW SHOULD CAUSAL CLAIMS BASED UPON THE RESULTS OF EPIDEMIOLOGIC RESEARCH BE WARRANTED?

Statistical inference and probability theory are central to epidemiologic research. The use of statistical applications in the analysis and interpretation of data are a fundamental aspect of epidemiologic methods [4]. Nevertheless, probabilistic relationships may be seen as surface phenomena of underlying causal mechanisms and relationships [18].

Approaches for warranting causal claims in epidemiology include quantitative models such as the counterfactual model and structural models—as discussed below—and qualitative approaches that rely more heavily on subject matter expertise (for example, background knowledge of environmental or chronic disease epidemiology), good judgment, and intuition. The Bradford Hill criteria for causal inference (or subsets or proposed refinements of the criteria) are widely used as a heuristic aid for assessing whether observed associations are causal. Examples of these causal criteria include the strength of an association, the specificity of an association, the consistency of an association across studies, and coherence or the extent to which a hypothesized causal association is compatible with preexisting theory and knowledge, and the temporal order [1]. A suspected causal factor must precede the effect or at least occur simultaneously. Criteria-based methods provide only general guidelines for assessing the causality of associations rather than a strict checklist for identifying a causal relationship [19]. Many exceptions can be cited to causal criteria and there are no "hard-and-fast rules of evidence" for assessing the causality of associations in epidemiologic research [20]. As a result, there has been increasing interest in developing quantitative approaches for identifying causal associations in epidemiologic research. Several quantitative approaches are discussed below.

QUANTITATIVE MODELS FOR IDENTIFYING CAUSAL ASSOCIATIONS

In recent decades, a rich literature has emerged on quantitative conceptual models for causal analysis in epidemiology, statistics, and the social sciences [18, 21-28]. The development of mathematical tools for identifying causal relationships in data has also helped to clarify assumptions needed to warrant causal claims. Proponents of causal modeling argue that, given certain assumptions, genuine causation can be distinguished from spurious covariation using computer algorithms, although not in every conceivable case. However, the notion of automating the discovery of causes using computer programs has been extensively debated by philosophers, computer scientists, and statisticians [2, 18, 29, 30].

Bayes-nets Methods. Bayes-nets methods, which have their roots in the probabilistic theory of causality, have been used (in fields other than epidemiology) for causal inference [2, 18]. Bayes-nets are directed acyclic graphs-as discussed by Pearl [18], Cartwright [2], and others-representing probabilistic independencies among an ordered set of variables. An example of a directed acyclic relationship between 2 variables is $X \rightarrow Y$. If X leads to Y and Y leads to X (i.e., $X \rightarrow Y$, $Y \rightarrow X$) then the directed relationship is cyclic. These methods have their metaphysical roots in the probabilistic theory of causality but Bayes-net methods act deterministically or at least quasi-deterministically [2]. Causal relationships are expressed in Bayes-nets in the form of deterministic, functional equations (i.e., equations in which a function is sought which satisfies certain relations among its values at all points). Probabilities are introduced through the assumption that certain variables in the equations are latent or unobserved [18]. These causal modeling frameworks are consistent with the view that "Nature possesses stable causal mechanisms that, on a detailed level of descriptions, are deterministic functional relationships between variables, some of which are unobservable" [18]. Baynes-net methods have several assumptions and limitations, for example, they do not apply to situations where the positive and negative effects of a factor cancel each other [2]. However, when the assumptions are met and the causal model is valid, much more information is provided than would be the case with statistical models.

To date, Bayes-nets methods have not been widely adopted for analyzing data from epidemiologic studies. Epidemiologists rely more heavily on study design, control of confounding variables, statistical analysis, and sound judgment for identifying and assessing causal relationships.

The Potential-Outcomes Model or Counterfactual Model. The potential-outcomes model or counterfactual model can be related both to graphical causal models (causal diagrams) and to structural-equation models [18]. Previous authors have described how the counterfactual theory of causation can be applied to observational data from epidemiologic or sociologic studies [23-27]. Counterfactual models specify what would happen under alternative possible patterns of exposure and provide a basis for quantitative analyses of exposure (or treatment) effects [24]. Statistical approaches to causal analysis require that the exposure of interest (X) and the outcome Y be measurable quantities [25].

Following the description provided by Greenland and Brumback [24], suppose that $i = 1,...,N$ represents a population of persons under study. The counterfactual model of causation assumes that: 1) each individual could have received any one of the exposure levels (or, in the context of a clinical trial, they could have been assigned to any treatment or comparison group at the time of random assignment), and 2) for each individual i and exposure level X_j, at the time of exposure (or random assignment of treatment), the outcome that individual i would have if the individual gets exposure level X_j exists, even if the individual does not actually get X_j. As discussed by Greenland and Brumback [24], this value is referred to as the potential outcome of individual i under exposure level X_j. The counterfactual model treats the potential outcome or outcomes as if they were baseline covariates or fixed from the start of follow-up [28].

The second assumption noted above can be restated in the following way: for each individual i and each exposure level X_j, a potential-outcome variable Y_{ij} can also be defined that represents the outcome of the individual under that exposure [24]. A further assumption in many counterfactual modeling applications is that the potential outcomes of each individual are independent of the exposures and outcomes of other individuals.

Y_{ij} is the indicator of the actual outcome for individual i if individual i has exposure level (or treatment) X_j. Otherwise, Y_{ij} may be quite different from the actual outcome [24]. This difference represents the effect of actual exposure level relative to exposure level X_j. The only Y_{ij} that can be observed is the one corresponding to the exposure actually received by individual i. As noted by Greenland and Brumback [24], the remaining Y_{ij} cannot be observed but they can be estimated from observed covariates and outcomes.

So far this discussion of causal analysis using the counterfactual model has focused on the situation where an individual is the study unit of interest. However, Greenland and Robins [28] explained that the counterfactual model can also be applied to situations where a cohort or population group is the study unit of interest:

"...the model encodes causal statements by assigning to each study unit (whether a person, cohort, or population) a different outcome variable for each exposure level. For a binary exposure indicator X, the familiar "Y" of associational (noncausal) regression analysis is replaced by a pair of variables Y_j, Y_0 representing the unit's outcome when exposed and the unit's outcome when not exposed, respectively: Y_1 is the outcome when X = 1, Y_0 is the outcome, when X = 0. Unit-level effects are differences or ratios of these exposure-specific and unit-specific outcomes" [28].

For multivariate treatments, where **X** is a vector, Y_x represents the outcome if **X** has specified values (denoted by x), i.e., where **X** = x.

Multiple causal factors can be taken into account in counterfactual models since causal factors may be necessary but not sufficient [25]. By specifying what would happen under alternative possible patterns of exposure, counterfactual models provide useful effect measures for etiologic studies [23]. This allows for the effect measure of interest (the causal contrast) to be more precisely defined than is sometimes the case in epidemiologic studies. A causal contrast compares disease frequency (in a particular target population during a specified time period) under two exposure distributions. A parameter that describes events under actual conditions is said to be actual or factual. In contrast, a parameter that describes events under a hypothetical alternative to actual conditions is counterfactual [23]. Counterfactual parameters cannot be observed since they describe hypothetical events following alternatives to actual conditions [23]. The exposure X should be a potentially changeable condition in order to make sense of the unobserved potential outcomes [27]. Counterfactual models can also specify probabilities or expected values for a potential outcome Y under a stochastic model and the model need not be deterministic [23].

Structural Equations Modeling. Structural equations modeling is a multivariate statistical technique in which a web or network of causation is modeled by a system of equations and independence assumptions [24, 31, 32]. Each equation shows how an individual response variable (outcome variable) changes as its direct causal variables change. As noted by Greenland and Brumback [24], "a variable may appear in no more than one equation as a response variable, but may appear in any other equation as a causal variable." In contrast to ordinary regression equations which represent associations of actual outcomes with actual values of covariates across individuals, structural equations may have within-individual causal interpretations [24]. Several authors have explicated the use of structural equations modeling in analyzing health data [18, 31, 32]. Specific examples from epidemiology were provided by Greenland and Brumback [24].

Structural equations modeling allows for the modeling of factors underlying multiple indicators of a construct and measurement error [33]. For example, Miller *et al.* [33] applied structural equations modeling to the analysis of data on combat exposures, PTSD symptoms, and global assessment of physical functioning in a sample of 315 Veterans seen at a Department of Veterans Affairs PTSD clinic [33]. Vasterling et al. [34] used structural equations modeling to evaluate the effect of PTSD on health-related function among U.S. Army soldiers who were assessed before and after deployments to Iraq. The study, which had a prospective design, was strengthened by the use of structural equations modeling and graphical models detailing the hypothesized structural models. The results showed that the severity of PTSD after deployment was associated with change in somatic health-related functioning and that postdeployment health symptoms is an intermediary variable [33].

Although structural equations have been extensively applied in psychology and other social sciences, social scientists do not always interpret results obtained from structural equations modeling as causal [18]. In addition, alternative approaches for causal modeling (for example, the potential-outcomes model or counterfactual model) have been preferred by some statisticians [18, 21]. Nevertheless, structural equation models can be linked to graphical causal models and causal diagrams [18, 24]. The use of structural equation models and causal diagrams to convey information about causal relationships offers an alternative to Bayesian methods which are used in such fields as medical decisionmaking and pharmacoepidemiology.

SUMMARY AND CONCLUSIONS

As Cartwright [2] noted, we are used to thinking of causation as one thing, even though we may accept that there are different methods to learn about it. If we also accept that there are different kinds of causation with different features (for example, deterministic and probabilistic causation), then we must consider which methods are appropriate for which kinds of causation [2]. This overview of quantitative models for identifying causal associations indicates that there are several approaches that are likely to be of use for epidemiologic research including structural equations modeling and the potential-outcomes model or counterfactual model. Both probabilistic and deterministic models of disease causation can be linked to sufficient-component models of disease causation. Outstanding questions include how best to apply probabilistic and deterministic models of disease causation into multilevel analyses, and whether Bayes-net methods have any utility for automating the discovery of the causes of illness and injuries in populations.

REFERENCES

[1]   Susser M. What is a cause and how do we know one? A grammar for pragmatic epidemiology. Am J Epidemiol 1991;133:635-48.

[2]   Cartwright N. Hunting Causes and Using Them. Approaches in Philosophy and Economics. New York: Cambridge University Press, 2007.

[3]   Popper KR. The Logic of Scientific Discovery. New York: Harper & Row, 1968.

[4]   Kleinbaum DG, Kupper LL, Morgenstern H. Epidemiologic Research: Principles and Quantitative Methods. Belmont, CA: Lifetime Learning Publications, 1982.

[5]   Buck C. Popper's philosophy for epidemiologists. Int J Epidemiol 1975;4:159-68.

[6]   Weed DL. On the logic of causal inference. Am J Epidemiol 1986;123:965-79.

[7]   Poole C. Induction does not exist in epidemiology. In: Rothman KJ, editor. Causal Inference. Chestnut Hill, MA: Epidemiology Resources, 1988; pp. 153-64.

[8]   Kuhn TS. Objectivity, value judgment, and theory choice. In: Kuhn TS, Ed. The Essential Tension. Chicago: University of Chicago Press, 1977; pp. 320-43.

[9]   Olsen J. What characterizes a useful concept of causation in epidemiology? J Epidemiol Commun Health 2003;57:86-88.

[10]   Karhausen LR. Causation: the elusive grail of epidemiology. Med Health Care Philos 2000;3:59-67.

[11]   Parascandola M, Weed DL. Causation in epidemiology. J Epidemiol Commun Health 2001;55:905-12.

[12]   Suppes P. A Probabilistic Theory of Causality. Amsterdam: North-Holland

Publishing Company, 1970.

[13]   Eells E. Probabilistic Causality. Cambridge, UK: Cambridge University Press, 1991.

[14]   Mackie JL. The Cement of the Universe. A Study of Causation. New York: Oxford University Press, 1974.

[15]   Hitchcock C. Probabilistic causation. In: Stanford Encyclopedia of Philosophy. Stanford, CA, 2002 http://plato.stanford.edu/entries/causation-probabilistic/.

[16]   Rothman KM. Causal inference in epidemiology. In: Modern Epidemiology. Boston: Little, Brown and Company, 1986.

[17]   Kaufman JS, Poole C. Looking back on "Causal Thinking in the Health Sciences." Ann Rev Public Health 2000;21:101-19.

[18]   Pearl J. Causality. New York: Springer, 2000.

[19]   Ward A. Causal criteria and the problem of complex causation. Med Health Care Philos 2009;12:333-43.

[20]   Rothman KJ, Greenland S. Causation and causal inference in epidemiology. Am J Public Health 2005;95:S144-S150.

[21]   Rubin DB. Estimating causal effects of treatments in randomized and nonrandomized studies. J Educ Psychol 1974;66:688-701.

[22]   Robins J, Greenland S. The probability of causation under a stochastic model for individual risk. Biometrics 1989;45:1125-38.

[23]   Maldonado G, Greenland S. Estimating causal effects. Int J Epidemiol 2002;31:422-9.

[24]   Greenland S, Brumback B. An overview of relations among causal modeling methods. Int J Epidemiol 2002;31:1030-7.

[25]   Hofler M. Causal inference based on counterfactuals. BMC Med Res Methodol 2005;5:28

[26]   Little RJ, Rubin DB. Causal effects in clinical and epidemiological studies via potential outcomes: concepts and analytical approaches. Annu Rev Public Health 2000;21:121-45.

[27]   Morgan SL, Winship C. Counterfactuals and Causal Inference. New York: Cambridge University Press, 2007.

[28]   Greenland S, Robins JM. Identifiability, exchangeability and confounding revisited. Epidemiologic Perspectives & Innovations 2009; pp. 6-4.

[29]   Aickin M. Causal Analysis in Biomedicine and Epidemiology. New York: Marcel Dekker, Inc., 2002.

[30]   Humphreys P, Freedman D. The grand leap. Br J Philos Sci 1996;47:113-23.

[31]   Goldeberg AS. Structural equation models in the social sciences. Econometrica 1972;40:979-1001.

[32]   Duncan OD. Introduction to Structural Equation Models. New York: Academic Press, 1975.

[33]   Miller MW, Wolf EJ, Martin E, *et al*. Structural equation modeling of associations among combat exposure, PTSD symptom factors, and Global Assessment of Functioning. J Rehabil Res Dev 2008;45:359-70.

[34]   Vasterling JJ, Schumm J, Proctor SP, *et al*. Posttraumatic stress disorder and health functioning in a non-treatment-seeking sample of Iraq war Veterans: a prospective analysis. J Rehabil Res Dev 2008;45:347-58.

CHAPTER 3

Seeking Causal Explanations in Epidemiology Subdisciplines

Abstract. Much of the literature on causal inference in epidemiologic research has dealt with causal inference in the field of epidemiology as a whole, or has focused on causal inference in certain areas such as chronic diseases and environmental causes of diseases and adverse health outcomes. In recent years, however, several authors have dealt with causal inference within a variety of epidemiologic subdisciplines including nutritional epidemiology, genetic epidemiology, infectious disease epidemiology, and social epidemiology. Although criteria-based approaches are still widely cited and used, enthusiasm for the Bradford Hill criteria or subsets of the criteria appears to be waning in some areas of epidemiology (or among some groups of epidemiologists). An increasing number of authors have argued that traditional criteria for causal inference in observational research do not apply to particular epidemiology subdisciplines or that certain criteria should be modified. A large and growing literature has dealt with quantitative models for estimating causal parameters using data from observational studies (for example, counterfactual models and structural equation models).

INTRODUCTION

A sizeable literature has accumulated on causal inference in epidemiology. Major approaches to causal inference in the field have included those based upon causal criteria or guidelines [1, 2], the sufficient component causes model [3, 4], and counterfactual models and other modeling approaches for causal inference from observational studies [5-9]. Much of the literature on causal inference in epidemiologic research has dealt with causal inference in the field of epidemiology as a whole, or has focused on causal inference in certain areas such as chronic diseases and environmental causes of diseases and adverse health outcomes. For example, the U.S. Environmental Protection Agency (EPA) Guidelines for Carcinogen Risk Assessment discuss a number of considerations in determining whether an association observed in epidemiologic research is causal or non-causal [10]. In recent years, however, several authors have dealt with causal inference within a variety of epidemiologic subdisciplines including nutritional epidemiology [11-13], genetic epidemiology [14], infectious disease epidemiology [15], pharmacoepidemiology [16, 17], and social epidemiology [18-24], as well as in viral carcinogenesis [25, 26]. An important question to consider is to what extent are methods and concepts for causal inference the same across epidemiologic subdisciplines? Or is it the case that certain approaches to causal inference or recent refinements are more likely to be applied within specific fields such as nutritional or genetic epidemiology? A related question is what

Steven S. Coughlin

kinds of refinements in approaches to causal inference are emerging within various subdisciplines and whether such refinements are suitable for other areas of epidemiology. Drawing upon the recent literature on causal inference in epidemiology, specific examples are provided below with the aim of summarizing recent developments in this area and drawing some conclusions about possible approaches for improving causal inference in the field.

BACKGROUND

As noted earlier in this volume, the 1964 Report of the Advisory Committee to the U.S. Surgeon General on "Smoking and Health" listed five criteria for evaluating the causality of an association: time order, strength, specificity, consistency, and coherence. In a summary of a lecture given to the Section of Occupational Medicine at the Royal Society of Medicine, Sir Austin Bradford Hill [1] expanded this list of criteria to include analogy, experimentation, and biologic gradient or dose-response curve. Bradford Hill also separated biologic plausibility from coherence. Susser [2] offered an account of what Bradford Hill meant by criteria such as analogy (which is infrequently invoked in practice) and experimentation and how sets of causal criteria have evolved over the half-century since Hill's now famous article was published. Causal criteria emphasized by Susser [2] include the strength of an association (the size of estimated risk), specificity (the precision with which one variable, to the exclusion of others, will predict the occurrence of another), consistency (the persistence of an association upon repeated test), predictive performance (the ability of a causal hypothesis drawn from an observed association to predict an unknown fact that is consequent on the initial association), and coherence (the extent to which a hypothesized causal association is compatible with preexisting theory and knowledge) [2]. In Susser's account, the presence of an association, time order (a suspected causal factor must precede the effect), and direction (change in an outcome is a consequence of change in an antecedent factor) are essential properties of causes rather than criteria for identifying causal associations like strength and consistency. The directionality of an association between exposure and a disease or other adverse health outcome is often an essential point in deliberations about the causality of an association.

The Bradford Hill criteria for causal inference or subsets of the criteria are still widely used as a heuristic aid for assessing whether associations observed in epidemiologic research are causal. For example, criteria or guidelines such as consistency, strength of the association, specificity, temporal relation, and biological plausibility were mentioned by the Global Advisory Committee on Vaccine Safety [27] and in the EPA Guidelines for Carcinogen Risk Assessment [10]. Rothman and Greenland [4] and other authors have noted that many exceptions can be cited to causal criteria and that there are no "hard-and-fast rules of evidence" for assessing the causality of associations in epidemiologic research. Criteria-based methods provide only general guidelines for assessing the causality of associations rather than a strict checklist for identifying a causal relationship [28].

Accounts of causal inference in epidemiology provided by Susser [2], Rothman [3], and others have pointed to the limitations of the Galilean concept of necessary and sufficient causes for elucidating the multiple causes of common and complex diseases and conditions which are often the focus of epidemiologic research today. Causes may be both necessary and sufficient to cause disease; they may be necessary but not sufficient; they may be sufficient but not necessary; or they may be neither necessary nor sufficient. In epidemiology, however, many causes of important diseases and health conditions are likely to be neither necessary nor sufficient.

The model of sufficient component causes proposed by Rothman [3] is widely used in epidemiology as a framework for understanding multicausality. A sufficient component cause is made up of a number of components, no one of which is sufficient for the disease or adverse health condition on its own [3, 4]. However, a sufficient cause exists when all the components are present. Diseases and adverse health conditions can be caused by more than one causal mechanism and each causal mechanism involves the combined action of several component causes. For example, mild traumatic brain injury may be the result of a fall, car accident, sports injury, or explosion or blast injury suffered during military service, and a variety of factors may interact to determine the extent of injury (for example, the nature of a physical impact or proximity to a blast, the availability of protective devices, genetic and biological factors, and the extent to which repetitive injuries occur over time). In Rothman's account, the apparent strength of a cause is determined by the prevalence of complimentary component causes. He convincingly argues that "the strength of an association is not a biologically consistent feature but rather a characteristic that depends on the relative prevalence of other causes" [3]. Interactions among component causes and induction and latency periods are also taken into account by Rothman's model. Although the model of sufficient component causes has much to recommend for conceptualizing multiple causes of a disease, some authors have argued that it does not sufficiently take into account the limited state of our knowledge about causal processes and that probabilistic definitions of causality are preferable [29, 30]. There is no consensus in the epidemiologic literature on whether a sufficient component model is the best conception of causation or whether other conceptual frameworks such as counterfactually-based statistical or probabilistic definitions of causation are preferable [30, 31].

In the discussion that follow, some developments in epidemiology subspecialties are considered with an eye toward identifying emerging approaches to causal inference including those that may be suitable for different areas of epidemiology. Finally, some suggestions are offered at the end about possible areas for further work on causal inference in epidemiology subdisciplines and in the field as a whole.

CAUSAL INFERENCE IN NUTRITIONAL EPIDEMIOLOGY

The field of nutritional epidemiology intersects with chronic disease epidemiology, environmental epidemiology, genetic epidemiology, and other epidemiologic subdisciplines. Like in other areas of epidemiology, causal inference is of great importance to the field. Previous authors have considered the criteria used to infer causality in observational or experimental studies of diet and nutrition in humans [11-13]. The Committee on Diet and Health of the National Research Council's Commission on Life Sciences evaluated the overall evidence for associations between nutrients, dietary patterns, and risk of chronic diseases (atherosclerotic cardiovascular diseases, cancer, diabetes, obesity, osteoporosis, dental caries, and chronic liver and kidney diseases) against six criteria. The latter included strength of association, dose-response relationship, temporally correct association, consistency of association, specificity of association, and biologic plausibility. All of these criteria were given roughly equal weight except for biologic plausibility. The Committee felt that biologic plausibility should be according somewhat less weight "since it is more dependent on subjective interpretation" [11]. While noting that the lack of a consensus on the role of diet in the etiology of chronic diseases partly stems from the absence of generally accepted criteria for interpreting the evidence, the Committee assessed the overall strength of the evidence from epidemiologic, clinical, and animal studies on a continuum from highly likely to very inconclusive. These assessments were partly based upon the overall strength and consistency of the data and the degree of concordance in evidence from epidemiologic, clinical, and laboratory studies. As part of their deliberations, the Committee considered the advantages and limitations of different types of studies (for example, epidemiologic studies with a case-control or prospective cohort study design, or randomized studies designed to test dietary interventions). The Committee concluded that "assessments of the strength of associations between diet and chronic diseases cannot simply be governed by criteria commonly used for inferring causality in other areas of human health" [11].

Potischman and Weed [13] outlined the causal criteria used in nutritional epidemiology to weigh the balance of benefits and risk associated with a nutrient or food. The causal criteria that they pointed to (based upon their understanding of the most commonly cited causal criteria in epidemiologic practice) includes consistency, strength of an association, dose response, biological plausibility, and temporality (correct temporal relationship), although they stopped short of arguing that every one of these should be met before a nutritional recommendation is made. In contrast to the Committee on Diet and Health [11], Potischman and Weed [13] did not cite specificity as a causal criterion nor did they consider evidence from intervention studies or from animal studies. Potischman and Weed noted that it would be difficult to make a case for consistency unless a majority of studies supported the nutritional hypothesis of interest, and that the assessment of consistency could be based upon studies restricted to those meeting certain standards of methodologic rigor. They further noted that, in nutritional epidemiology, such assessments of the consistency of study findings may be complicated by measurement error, lack of variation of food or nutrient intake in the population, and the lack of comparability of some dietary assessment tools. In their account, "a statistically significant risk estimate that is a >20% increase or decrease in risk is considered a positive finding," which reflects the fact that evidence of weak associations or null findings are a frequent occurrence in nutritional epidemiology [13].

In addition to identifying a set of causal criteria likely to be of value in nutritional epidemiology, Potischman and Weed called for "a clear description of the rules of inference used for each criterion, i.e., the types or extent of evidence needed to meet that criterion" [13]. However, they acknowledged that there is no strong consensus in the field about the relative importance of causal criteria or about the rules of inference that should be assigned to any particular criterion. In addition to causal inference based upon criteria, Potischman and Weed pointed out the importance of a variety of scientific considerations in reaching judgments about nutrition recommendations, including study designs, statistical tests, bias, confounding, and the quality of measurements [13]. Similar considerations had been pointed to by Susser in his early work on causal thinking in the health sciences.

Another account of causal inference in nutritional epidemiology was provided by Willett [12] who noted that true associations are not likely to be strong in nutritional studies although relative risks in the range of 0.7 or 1.5 could potentially be important because many dietary exposures are common. Willet also highlighted the fact that dose-response relationships are often nonlinear and null findings may occur even when a causal relationship exists, i.e., absolute consistency across studies is an unrealistic expectation in nutritional epidemiology. Also of interest is Willett's account of the evaluation of null or statistically non-significant findings in studies of diet and disease. For example, a relationship could go undetected because the approach taken to measure dietary intake may not be sufficiently precise, the variation in diet may be insufficiently great in the study population, or the temporal relationship between the measured exposure and the occurrence of disease does not encompass the latent period [12].

More recently, authors have discussed methodological issues related to causal inference using associations with body mass index as an example but the focus is on methods for epidemiology as a whole rather than nutritional epidemiology (or chronic disease epidemiology) in particular [32].

CAUSAL INFERENCE IN GENETIC EPIDEMIOLOGY

Ioannidis *et al.* [14] noted that guidelines for inferring causation in observational studies have been modified for various fields in epidemiology. They argued that established guides for causal inference in epidemiology are inappropriate for assessing genetic associations such as those identified in genome-wide association studies where associations with hundreds of thousands of genetic variants may be examined [14]. Temporality is not an important consideration for genetic factors fixed at birth, although epi-genetic influences may transcend generations. Because of gene-environment interactions and other factors, the existence and strength of genetic associations may vary across populations and weak associations are frequently identified. In many epidemiologic studies, weak causal effects are often difficult to distinguish from non-causal associations that are due to methodological biases. To overcome such limitations of traditional causal criteria, Ioannidis *et al.* [14] proposed a semi-quantitative index that assigns three levels for the amount of evidence, extent of replication, and protection from bias. Following this approach, a composite assessment of strong, moderate, or weak epidemiologic *credibility* of a genetic association is obtained. Ioannidis *et al.* used the term credibility to refer to the likelihood than an association exists after some evidence has been accumulated. In their account, the credibility of a genetic association is improved by consistent evidence such as that obtained "by virtue of many studies, or by a more modest number of large studies." However, the consistency argument is weakened by the fact that gene-environment interactions are known to occur. The credibility of a genetic association is increased by evidence from a well-conducted meta-analysis showing a consistent association and little heterogeneity across study populations. Similar approaches have been used to grade the quality of evidence for the effectiveness of medical interventions [33]. A potential disadvantage of the use of semi-quantitative indices to assess genetic associations is that they currently do not assess the concordance of biological and epidemiological evidence.

Of course, these are not the only authors who have dealt with methodological issues in genetic epidemiology that have potential implications for causal inference. For example, a recent article by VanderWeele *et al.* [34] on case-only gene-environment interaction studies can be tied to the sufficient component causes model of causation. The methodological literature in genetics, and epidemiology as a whole, continues to move forward very rapidly and further important developments are inevitable.

CAUSAL INFERENCE IN INFECTIOUS DISEASE EPIDEMIOLOGY AND VIRAL CARCINOGENESIS

Another epidemiology subdiscipline that has strived to develop refined criteria for inferring causation is infectious disease epidemiology, partly because of the intersecting field of viral carcinogenesis. Kosch's postulates and later refinements have long provided a framework to readily identify acute diseases associated with microorganisms [36]. The deterministic criteria for causality proposed by Robert Koch applied tests to identify causative agents of infectious disease. For example, the agent must always be found with the disease, the agent must be shown by isolation and culture to be a living organism and distinct from any other that might be found with the disease, and the agent, isolated from the body in pure culture, must induce the disease in susceptible experimental animals. Koch's first postulate, that an infectious agent must always be found with the disease, is relevant when a disease is defined on the basis of the presence of the agent.

In contemporary infectious disease epidemiology, causal modeling of disease data (both direct and indirect effects) are often of interest including changes in susceptibility and changes in infectiousness [15]. Such direct and indirect effects are linked by transmission probabilities. In infectious disease transmission, whether a person becomes infected depends upon who else is infected [15, 35]. Related methodologic topics, such as control of confounding and measurement issues in studies of vaccine effectiveness, have been addressed in the recent literature, but those topics are beyond the scope of the present review.

Infectious disease epidemiology overlaps with chronic disease and genetic epidemiology since infectious agents have been implicated in the etiology of certain forms of cancer [26, 37]. Both the Bradford Hill criteria for causal inference and the Evans' modified guidelines have been used to evaluate associations between viruses and cancer [25]. In their summary of an expert workshop having to do with criteria for establishing human cancer etiology, Carbone et al. [26] argued that "A few of the Hill's criteria have not stood the test of time and cannot be considered essential: specificity, analogy, plausibility, and coherence." They also noted that over the past decade, epidemiologic methods have been increasingly integrated with the methods of molecular pathology in order to more rapidly and accurately identify human carcinogens [26]. Findings from molecular pathology and laboratory studies may help to identify carcinogens more rapidly such as when long latency periods are needed to identify causal associations in epidemiologic studies of infectious agents.

CAUSAL INFERENCE IN PHARMACOEPIDEMIOLOGY

Pharmacoepidemiology involves the application of epidemiological methods and concepts to study the effects of drugs in large populations [16, 17]. The methods of pharmacoepidemiology and pharmacovigiliance are used to monitor, detect, and evaluate adverse effects of medications during the postmarketing period. Based upon the Bradford Hill criteria, Strom [16] provided a summary of criteria for the causal nature of an association in the third edition of his well-known text on *Pharmacoepidemiology*. The criteria cited by Strom included coherence with existing information (biological plausibility), consistency of the association, time sequence, specificity of the association, and strength of the association. In Strom's account, the strength of the association is related to the quantitative strength of an association and whether there is a dose-response relationship. Strom also related the strength of an association to aspects of study design (the type of study design used in the studies in question and whether they were well-designed) which other authors have related to the strength or quality of a body of scientific evidence [33, 38]. Strom noted that no one of the criteria is absolutely necessary for an association to be causal in nature and that no one of them is sufficient for an association to be considered a causal association. The more criteria that are satisfied, the more likely it is that an association is a causal association [16]. Strom argued that coherence "refers to whether the association makes sense, in light of other types of information available in the literature" (data from other studies involving humans, data from animal studies, data from in vitro research, and scientific or pathophysiologic theory). With respect to the consistency of an association, he noted that reproducibility is a hallmark of science. Specifically, "if a finding is real, one should be able to reproduce it in a different setting" [16]. In Strom's account, the criterion of specificity (whether the cause ever occurs without the presumed effect and whether the effect occurs without the presumed cause) is "almost never met in biology, with the occasional exception of infectious diseases" [16]. Finally, Strom noted that "A dose-response relationship is an extremely important and commonly used concept in clinical pharmacology and is used similarly in epidemiology" [16].

While emphasizing the value of the Bradford-Hill criteria for causal inference in pharmacoepidemiology, Shakir and Layton [17] argued that with marketed medicines it is rare to find relative risks greater than 2.0 for adverse drug reactions. Although not everyone would agree with that claim, it is certainly true that methods for evaluating weak associations (i.e., those with a relative risk less than 2.0) are also needed in pharmacoepidemiology [16, 17].

Criteria such as strength of the association, consistency, specificity, temporal relation, and biological plausibility have also been used to assess the causality of adverse events following immunization [27]. However, not all of these criteria need to be satisfied for a causal relationship between an adverse event and a vaccine to be present [27].

In addition to accounts of causal inference in pharmacoepidemiology [16, 17], a sizeable literature has accumulated on approaches for determining the causality of adverse reactions from drugs or vaccines from case reports or case series [39, 40-44]. This literature, which runs parallel to the literature on causal inference in pharmacoepidemiology and other epidemiology subdisciplines, includes algorithms, diagrams, decision tables, and probabilistic or Bayesian approaches for evaluating the causality of adverse reactions from case reports [41-43, 45]. Case reports and case series can provide useful information about adverse drug effects when outcomes among exposed individuals are dramatically different from what one might expect among nonexposed individuals. Although there are some similarities between the evaluation of causality in case reports and causal inference in epidemiology, there are also some notable differences [39]. For example, the context of adverse reaction assessment is often an individual clinical event or a small number of adverse events suspected of being associated with a drug or vaccine and there may be an opportunity to obtain additional pharmacologic evidence, for example, the result of withdrawing the drug ("dechallenge") and the result of reintroducing the drug ("rechallenge"). Adverse reactions can be acute or chronic, reversible or not, rare or common, and can be identical to well-characterized common diseases (for example, myocardial infarction) or pathologically unique [39].

In addition to the above accounts of causal inference in pharmacoepidemiology, several authors have addressed related methodological issues such as the use of instrumental variables [6, 46-48] and the use of propensity score approaches to control for confounding in epidemiologic research [49-54]. However, the use of propensity scores to control for confounding extends beyond observational pharmacoepidemiologic research.

CAUSAL INFERENCE IN SOCIAL EPIDEMIOLOGY

Social epidemiology is a further epidemiologic subdiscipline that has witnessed vigorous discussion and debate about aspects of causal inference. For example Susser and Schwartz [18] argued that social characteristics (for example, race) should not be singled out "as posing an especially severe problem for causal inference." Their arguments were in response to questions raised by Greenland [55] about whether socioeconomic indicators of disease should be viewed as causes. An earlier discussion of causal explanations in social epidemiology also revolved around important issues such as whether race should be viewed as a risk factor and the extent to which various mechanisms of disease causation account for health disparities [19, 21].

Other important topics dealt with in the literature on causal inference in social epidemiology include applications of the counterfactual causal framework to multilevel health research [20] and the use of structural equations modeling and path analysis to illuminate social mechanisms of disease causation [22, 56]. The literature on causal inference in social epidemiology [18-22] can be related to the even larger literature on epidemiologic paradigms and theories of disease causation [57-60] as discussed elsewhere in this volume.

SUMMARY AND CONCLUSIONS

This review of the literature on causal inference in epidemiology subdisciplines indicates that there are notable differences in the extent to which epidemiologists support the use of criterion-based approaches such as the Bradford Hill criteria or sets of criteria based upon the criteria proposed by Bradford Hill. Although criteria-based approaches are still widely cited and used in such fields as environmental and occupational epidemiology, chronic disease epidemiology, and pharmacoepidemiology, enthusiasm for the Bradford Hill criteria or subsets of the criteria appears to be waning in some areas of epidemiology (or among some groups of epidemiologists). In fields as diverse as nutritional epidemiology and genetic epidemiology, an increasing number of authors have argued that all or at least some traditional criteria for causal inference in observational research do not apply or that certain criteria should be modified (for example, to assist with the identification of weak causal associations where odds ratios or relative risk estimates may be less than 2.0). Of course, weak associations may be of interest in any area of epidemiology and are not unique to certain subdisciplines. Nevertheless, some authors have implied that weak associations and null findings are especially common in nutritional epidemiology. Hernan and Cole [32] recently discussed the issue of how substantial measurement error affects causal inference in epidemiology.

In the field of epidemiology as a whole, there appears to be widespread appreciation of the fact that causal criteria do not provide strict guidelines for assessing the causality of associations identified in epidemiologic studies and hence should not be viewed as a "checklist" of criteria that must be satisfied in order for an association to be causal. Not only do causal criteria or guidelines serve only as a general guide for thinking about the causality of associations observed in observational research, they form "but one of five strategies Susser originally described for coming to judgments about causality from epidemiologic results. The other four were to simplify the conditions of observation in study design and execution, to screen for confounders analytically, to elaborate associations analytically, and to use significance test and power analyses to address the role of chance." [24]. To overcome limitations of traditional causal criteria, and to allow for the identification of weak but potentially important associations, some investigators are focusing on the amount of evidence and protection from bias rather than the strength of the association per se. A focus on evaluating competing causal theories using crucial observations may also be helpful [4]. There have been calls for more realistic assessments of the consistency of associations across studies.

A potential limitation of this review is that it does not summarize the literature on causal inference in all epidemiologic subdisciplines or related fields. For example, the current review does not deal with causal inference in clinical epidemiology or reproductive epidemiology. In addition, a large and growing literature has dealt with quantitative models for estimating causal parameters using data from observational studies (for example, counterfactual models and structural equation models) as reviewed elsewhere in this volume. Such approaches require making several assumptions and, like with alternative approaches to causal inference, they do not allow for causal hypotheses to be proven [5, 6, 8, 9].

Possible areas for further work include empirical studies to consider whether statistical approaches for causal analysis of data from observational studies [5, 6, 8, 9] are suitable for specific epidemiologic subdisciplines. For example, do such modeling approaches work equally well for nutritional and genetic epidemiology or are they mostly applicable to other areas of epidemiology such as chronic disease or environmental epidemiology? Similarly, work done to apply Bayesian techniques to specific topics (for example, surveillance of drug adverse effects) could be extended to other epidemiologic subdisciplines. Additional suggestions for further work in this area are offered in the concluding chapter in this volume.

REFERENCES

[1]   Hill AB, 1965. The environment and disease: association or causation? Proc R Soc Med 1965;58:295-300.

[2]   Susser M. What is a cause and how do we know one? A grammar for pragmatic epidemiology. Am J Epidemiol 1991;133:635-48.

[3]   Rothman KM. Causal inference in epidemiology. In: Modern Epidemiology. Boston: Little, Brown and Company, 1986.

[4]   Rothman KJ, Greenland S. Causation and causal inference in epidemiology. Am J Public Health 2005;95:S144-S150.

[5]   Greenland S. An overview of methods for causal inference from observational studies. In: Gelman A, Meng XL, Eds. Applied Bayesian Modeling and Causal Inference from An Incomplete-data Perspective. New York: Wiley, 2004.

[6]   Greenland S. Causal analysis in the health sciences. J Am Stat Assoc 2000;95:286-9.

[7]   Greenland S, Brumback B. An overview of relations among causal modeling

methods. Int J Epidemiol 2002;31:1030-7.

[8]   Little RJ, Rubin DB. Causal effects in clinical and epidemiological studies via potential outcomes: concepts and analytical approaches. Ann Rev Public Health 2000;21:121-45.

[9]   Robins JM, Greenland S. The probability of causation under a stochastic model for individual risks. Biometrics 1989;45:112538.

[10]   Environmental Protection Agency. Notice of Availability of the Document Entitled Guidelines for Carcinogen Risk Assessment. Federal Register April 7, 2005, vol. 70, pp. 17765-817. http://www.epa.gov/EPA~RESEARCH/2005/April/Day~07/r6642.htm.

[11]   Committee on Diet and Health, National Research Council. Diet and Health: Implications for Reducing Chronic Disease Risk. Washington, DC: National Academy Press, 1989.

[12]   Willett W. Nutritional Epidemiology, 2nd Ed. New York: Oxford University Press, 1998.

[13]   Potischman N, Weed DL. Causal criteria in nutritional epidemiology. Am J Clin Nutr 1999;69:1309S-14S.

[14]   Ioannidis JP, Boffetta P, Little J, *et al*. Assessment of cumulative evidence on genetic associations: interim guidelines. Int J Epidemiol 2008;37:120-32.

[15]   Halloran ME, Struchiner CJ. Causal inference in infectious diseases. Epidemiology 1995;6:142-51.

[16]   Strom BL, Ed. Pharmacoepidemiology, 3rd ed. Chichester: Wiley and Sons Ltd., 2000.

[17]   Shakir SAW, Layton D. Causal association in pharmacovigilance and pharmacoepidemiology. Thoughts on the application of the Austin Bradford-Hill criteria. Drug Safety 2002:25:467-71.

[18]   Susser E, Schwartz S. Are social causes so different from all other causes? A comment on Sander Greenland. Emerg Themes Epidemiol 2005;2:4.

[19]   Kaufman JS, Cooper RS. Seeking causal explanations in social epidemiology. Am J Epidemiol 1999;150:113-20.

[20]   Oakes JM. The (mis)estimation of neighborhood effects: causal inference for a practicable social epidemiology. Social Sci Med 2004;58:1929-52.

[21]   Muntaner C. Social mechanisms, race, and social epidemiology. Am J Epidemiol 1999;150:121-8.

[22]   Hafeman DM, Schwartz S. Opening the black box: a motivation for the assessment of mediation. Int J Epidemiol 2009:38:838-45.

[23]   Kaufman JS, Poole C. Looking back on "Causal Thinking in the Health

Sciences." Ann Rev Public Health 2000;21:101-19.

[24]   Susser M. Causal Thinking in the Health Sciences: Concepts and Strategies of Epidemiology. New York: Oxford University Press, 1973.

[25]   Evans AS, Mueller NE. Viruses and cancer causal associations. Ann Epidemiol 1990;1:71-92.

[26]   Carbone M, Klein G, Gruber J, Wong M. Modern criteria to establish human cancer etiology. Cancer Res 2004;64:5518-24.

[27]   World Health Organization Global Advisory Committee on Vaccine Safety. Causality assessment of adverse events following immunization. http://www.who.int/vaccine_safety/causality/en/

[28]   Ward A. Causal criteria and the problem of complex causation. Med Health Care Philos 2009;12:333-43.

[29]   Kleinbaum DG, Kupper LL, Morgenstern H. Epidemiologic Research: Principles and Quantitative Methods. Belmont, CA: Lifetime Learning Publications, 1982.

[30]   Parascandola M, Weed DL. Causation in epidemiology. J Epidemiol Commun Health 2001;55:905-12.

[31]   Olsen J. What characterizes a useful concept of causation in epidemiology? J Epidemiol Commun Health 2003;57:86-88.

[32]   Hernan MA, Cole SR. Causal diagrams and measurement bias. Am J Epidemiol 2009;170:959-62.

[33]   Atkins D, Best D, Briss PA, *et al.* Grading quality of evidence and strength of recommendations. Br Med J 2004;328:1490.

[34]   VanderWeele TJ, Hernandez-Diaz S, Hernan MA. Case-only gene-environment interaction studies: when does association imply mechanistic interaction? Genetic Epidemiol 2010;34:327-34.

[35]   Hudgens MG, Halloran ME. Toward causal inference with interference. J Am Stat Assoc 2008;103:832-42.

[36]   Evans AS. Causation and disease: the Henle-Koch postulates revisited. Yale J Biol Med 1976;50:175-95.

[37]   McNicholl JM, Cuenco KT. Host genes and infectious diseases. HIV, other pathogens, and a public health perspective. Am J Prev Med 1999;16:141-54.

[38]   Lohr KN. Rating the strength of scientific evidence: relevance for quality improvement programs. Int J Qual Health Care 2004;16:9-18.

[39]   Jones JK. Determining causation from case reports. In: Strom BL, editor. Pharmacoepidemiology, 3rd ed. Chichester: Wiley and Sons Ltd., 2000.

[40]   Irey NS. Adverse drug reactions and death: a review of 827 cases. JAMA 1976;236:575-8.

[41]   Lane DA. A probabilist's view of causality assessment. Drug Inf J 1984;18:323-30.

[42]   Lance DA, Kramer MS, Hutchinson TA, et al. The causality assessment of adverse drug reactions using a Bayesian approach. Pharm Med 1987;2:265-83.

[43]   Jones JK. A Bayesian approach to causality assessment. Psychopharmacol Bull 1987;23:395-9.

[44]   Karch FE, Lasagna L. Toward the operational identification of adverse drug reactions. Clin Pharmacol Ther 1977;21:247-54.

[45]   Lance D. Causality assessment for adverse drug reactions: a probabilistic approach. In: Berry D, Ed. Statistical Methodology in the Pharmaceutical Sciences. New York: Dekker, 1990.

[46]   Martens EP, Pestman WR, de Boer A, *et al*. Instrumental variables. Application and limitations. Epidemiology 2006;17:260-7.

[47]   Hernan MA, Robins JM. Instruments for causal inference. An epidemiologist's dream? Epidemiology 2006;17:360-72.

[48]   Hogan JW, Lancaster T. Instrumental variables and inverse probability weighting for causal inference from longitudinal observational studies. Stat Methods Med Res 2004;13:17-48.

[49]   Hansen BB. The essential role of balance tests in propensity-matched observational studies: Comments on 'A critical appraisal of propensity-score matching in the medical literature between 1996 and 2003' by Peter Austin. Stat Med 2008;27:2050-4.

[50]   Austin PC. The performance of different propensity score methods for estimating marginal odds ratios. Stat Med 2007;26:3078-94.

[51]   Austin PC. The performance of different propensity-score methods for estimating relative risks. J Clin Epidemiol 2008;61:537-45.

[52]   Stuart EA. Developing practical recommendations for the use of propensity scores: discussion of 'A critical appraisal of propensity score matching in the medical literature between 1996 and 2003' by Peter Austin. Stat Med 2008;27:2062-5.

[53]   Shah BR, Laupacis A, Hux JE, Austin PC. Propensity score methods gave similar results to traditional regression modeling in observational studies: a systematic review. J Clin Epidemiol 2005;58:550-9.

[54]   Sturmer T, Joshi M, Glynn RJ, Avorn J, *et al*. A review of the application of

propensity score methods yielded increasing use, advantages in specific settings, but not substantially different estimates compared with conventional multivariable methods. J Clin Epidemiol 2006;59:437-47.

[55]   Greenland S. Epidemiologic measures and policy formulation: lessons from potential outcomes. Emerg Themes Epidemiol 2005;2:5

[56]   Factor-Litvak P, Sher A. Coming out of the box. Am J Epidemiol 2009;169:1179-81.

[57]   Susser M, Susser E. Choosing a future for epidemiology: II. From black box to Chinese Boxes and eco-epidemiology. Am J Public Health 1996;86:674-7.

[58]   Krieger N. Epidemiology and the web of causation: has anyone seen the spider? Soc Sci Med 1994;39:887-903.

[59]   Coughlin SS. Scientific paradigms in epidemiology and professional values. Epidemiology 1998;9:578-80.

[60]   McMichael AJ. Prisoners of the proximate: loosening the constraints on epidemiology in an age of change. Am J Epidemiol 1999;149:887-97.

CHAPTER 4

Scientific Paradigms in Epidemiology and Professional Values

Abstract. A notable feature of the debate about scientific paradigms and theories in epidemiology has been the juxtaposition of scientific, social, and ethical arguments. In some articles on epidemiologic theory and scientific paradigms, ethical issues and professional values have been discussed in order to bolster or clarify the authors' scientific arguments or to point to future directions. However, the introduction of statements laden with social concerns, ethics, and values into a scientific discussion of epidemiologic theory tends to obscure the scientific issues at the heart of the debate. Analyses of professional values and ethics in epidemiology are vitally important, but they should be thorough and well balanced and clearly distinguished as considerations of ethical and social concerns. Judgments about the relative *scientific* merits of alternative scientific paradigms (or proposed refinements in existing paradigms) should be based upon scientific considerations.

INTRODUCTION

The lively debate about scientific paradigms and theories in epidemiology has drawn attention to differences in perspectives about scientific frameworks in the field [1-10]. A notable feature of this debate has been the juxtaposition of scientific, social, and ethical arguments. For example, in addition to methodologic and scientific shortcomings, critics of "risk factor epidemiology" have cited the potential for persons with disease to be unfairly blamed for their illness [7, 11]. They have argued that research strategies that focus exclusively on individual behaviors such as cigarette smoking and high-risk sexual practices and that fail to take into account social and environmental determinants of health and disease may lead to "victim blaming." In three articles on epidemiologic theory and scientific paradigms, ethical issues and professional values have been discussed as concluding remarks, to bolster or clarify the authors' scientific arguments or to point to future directions [6, 9, 10].

Susser and Susser [6] argued for a more "humane" discipline in calling for a paradigm shift from the current emphasis on individual risk factors for disease to a new ecologic approach (a "Chinese boxes paradigm" or "eco-epidemiology"), which encompasses many levels of organization, including molecular, individual, and societal. The implication is that the prevailing paradigm or "black box epidemiology" (relating exposures to disease outcome without necessarily identifying intervening factors or pathogenesis) is less humane and therefore less defensible from an ethical standpoint. At the end of their far-ranging commentary about the future of epidemiology, Susser and Susser underscored the importance of professional and "ethical obligations for service to individuals or society," "social equity," and the need for a return to "public health values" [6].

In an article defending the need for epidemiologic theory [which they had previously defined as "interconnected ideas about what explains population health"[4], Krieger and Zierler [9] cautioned "that application of some frameworks may be morally untenable." They upheld Richard Levins' view that "all theories are wrong which promote, justify, or tolerate injustice" [12]. Krieger and Zierler noted that, as epidemiologists, they share in a vision of reducing human suffering through the generation of beneficial knowledge [9].

It is hard not to be moved by such deeply felt humanitarian concerns. Nevertheless, the introduction of statements laden with social concerns, ethics, and values into a scientific discussion of epidemiologic theory tends to obscure the scientific issues at the heart of the debate. For example, in a commentary about "black box epidemiology," Weed [10] argued that epidemiologists "need a common set of moral values" and that they lack a consensus about their obligation to public health. He concluded that "there is a need to explicate and to agree on the basic values of the discipline" in order to move the debate about scientific paradigms forward [10]. Echoing Susser and Susser's concern over the need to socialize public health students to "common values" [6], Weed argued for reaching agreement upon "a common set of moral values," with the goal of mending "conceptual rifts" about scientific paradigms and bringing about an end to "professional incohesiveness" in the field [10]. Weed's scientific arguments about alternative paradigms in epidemiology ("epidemiologists should embrace rather than denigrate the idea of black boxes" [10, p. 13] and "epidemiologists should get beyond the pejorative connotation of black box thinking by embracing a systems theory approach while remaining aware of its weaknesses" [10, p. 14]) are partly obscured by his repeated appeals to "moral values" and by the metaphors for morally dubious agents that abound in his commentary (for example, "divisive forces," "divide and conquer," and "socio-political forces")[10].

Will paying more attention to core values clarify or end the debate about scientific paradigms? Simply put, core values in epidemiology are basic scientific values internal to the profession that reflect and provide support for the mission and purpose of epidemiology. As Gellermann *et al.* [13] explained, core values reflect what the profession stands for, what it intends to promote through its work, and what its members aspire toward. Although differences of opinion about core values may well exist in the field [14-16], it is not clear that reaching a consensus about core values would resolve the scientific debate over alternative scientific paradigms and theories in epidemiology. Some of the differences of opinion may lie, not in core values, but rather in further specifications of less fundamental ethical rules and professional norms, such as how best to communicate valid scientific information that can be used to protect public health or formulate sound public health policy [17-19]. Moreover, many epidemiologists, including those in subspecialty areas such as clinical epidemiology and molecular epidemiology, may share Krieger and Zierler's [4] Susser and Susser's [6], and Pearce's [7] affinity for public health values. Those who don't may contribute to the profession in other important ways.

The concern over commonality of values [6, 10] is misplaced in the midst of a scientific debate. Diversity of values is likely to be beneficial to a relatively young and still-evolving profession like epidemiology. Like scientific theories and paradigms, core values within epidemiology and other professions may evolve over time, and more than one set of values may be upheld, especially during periods of transition.

Another potential problem with the introduction of statements about ethics and values into a scientific discourse is that it may fail to give the ethical and social issues the attention they deserve. Analyses of professional values and ethics in epidemiology are vitally important, but these should be thorough and well balanced and clearly distinguished as considerations of ethical and social concerns.

All scientific paradigms and theories have the potential to raise ethical and social concerns. For example, the acceptance of the germ theory of disease causation around the turn of the last century raised new ethical concerns related to personal autonomy and the potential for disease transmission [20]. In recent years, new ethical and social concerns have arisen as a result of advances in molecular genetics and molecular epidemiology that require careful analysis [21-24]. Although "risk factor epidemiology" has raised concerns about the stigmatization of risk groups and communities [25, 26], the extent to which alternative theoretical frameworks in epidemiology pose risks and harms or fail to ensure an equitable distribution of risks and potential benefits has not been carefully analyzed.

An eco-epidemiology" approach, as proposed by Susser and Susser [5, 6], would presumably require the use of extensive health information systems and sharpen concerns about personal privacy and confidentiality of health information [27, 28]. Justice-related concerns can also be raised since some developing countries might lack the necessary public health infrastructure to benefit fully from an eco-epidemiology approach. of course, this concern might also apply to alternative scientific paradigms in epidemiology.

Advances in genetics may require the reframing of the debate over "risk factor epidemiology"-including the extent to which it leads to "victim blaming." For example, an editorial about the DRD2 gene, smoking, and lung cancer [29] asked: "Why do some individuals smoke and others do not? Why can some smokers quit, while others cannot? Why do certain smokers develop cancer of the lung, while others, despite prolonged use of cigarettes, do not?" Genetic factors explain why some individuals infected with the human immunodeficiency virus (HIV) do not progress to AIDS [30]. Nevertheless, an improved understanding of how genes contribute to cancer, AIDS, and other diseases for which the sick have sometimes been unfairly blamed is unlikely to do away with concerns about personal (or societal) responsibility for smoking, HIV infection, or other factors that interact with genetic susceptibility factors for disease. Moreover, the acceptance of a new scientific paradigm in epidemiology that de-emphasizes individual risk factors for disease may simply shift part of the blame for illness from personal behaviors to "bad genes," which have themselves been associated with social stigma and discrimination [31, 32].

Philosophers and historians of science have often observed that social concerns and values influence the conduct and interpretation of scientific research [33-35]. It does not follow from these observations, however, that epidemiologists and other scientists should stop striving to separate clearly scientific and nonscientific considerations. Nor does it follow that epidemiologists should disclose their values in scientific articles—or encourage others to do so [36]—to allow others to better evaluate their scientific conclusions. The important issue, from a scientific perspective, is whether the theory is valid or useful, not what the values of the theorist are. Encouraging epidemiologists to disclose their values in scientific articles is yet another example of judging authors rather than their words [37]. The philosophical and historical evidence that science is not value-free does indicate that scientific, social, and ethical arguments should be mixed with caution.

On balance, it seems prudent not to juxtapose questions of social concerns, values, and ethics with scientific considerations in debating the strengths and weaknesses of alternative scientific paradigms and theories. Judgments about the relative *scientific* merits of alternative scientific paradigms (or proposed refinements in existing paradigms) should be based upon scientific considerations.

REFERENCES

[1]   Savitz DA. In defense of black box epidemiology. Epidemiology 1994;5:550-2.

[2]   Skrabanek P. The emptiness of the black box. Epidemiology 1994;5:553-5.

[3]   Krieger N. Epidemiology and the web of causation: has anyone seen the spider? Soc Sci Med 1994;39:887-903.

[4]   Krieger N, Zierler S. What explains the public's health: a call for epidemiologic theory. Epidemiology 1995;7:107-9.

[5]   Susser M, Susser E. Choosing a future for epidemiology. I. Eras and paradigms. Am J Public Health 1996;86:668-73.

[6]   Susser M, Susser E. Choosing a future for epidemiology. II. From black box to Chinese boxes and eco-epidemiology. Am J Public Health 1996;86:674-7.

[7]   Pearce N. Traditional epidemiology, modern epidemiology, and public health. Am J Public Health 1996;86:678-83.

[8]   Savitz DA. The alternative to epidemiologic theory: whatever works. Epidemiology 1997;8:210-12.

[9]   Krieger N, Zierler S. The need for epidemiologic theory. Epidemiology 1997;8:212-4.

[10]   Weed DL. Beyond black box epidemiology. Am J Public Health 1998;88:12-14.

[11]   McKinlay JB. Towards appropriate levels of analysis, research methods and health public policy. Presented at the International Symposium on Quality of Life and Health: Theoretical and Methodological Considerations, Berlin, May 25-27, 1994.

[12]   Levins R. Ten propositions on science and antiscience. Soc Text 1996;46/47:101-11.

[13]   Gellermann W, Frankel MS, Ladenson RF. Values and Ethics in Organization and Human Systems Development: Responding to Dilemmas in Professional Life. San Francisco: Jossey-Bass, 1990.

[14]   Coughlin SS. Ethics in epidemiology and public health practice. In: Coughlin SS, Ed. Ethics in Epidemiology and Public Health Practice: Collected Works. Columbus, GA: Quill Publications, 1997: 9-26.

[15] Weed DL. Science, ethics guidelines, and advocacy in epidemiology. Ann Epidemiol 1994;4:166-71.

[16] Coughlin SS. Advancing professional ethics in epidemiology. J Epidemiol Biostat 1996;1:71-77.

[17] Schulte PA, Singal M. Ethical issues in the interaction with subjects and disclosure of results. In: Coughlin SS, Beauchamp TL, Eds. Ethics and Epidemiology. New York: Oxford University Press, 1996; pp. 178-96.

[18] Sandman PM. Emerging communication responsibilities of epidemiologists. J Clin Epidemiol 1991;44(Suppl I):41S-50S.

[19] Rothman KJ, Poole C. Science and policymaking (editorial). Am J Public Health 1985;75:340-1.

[20] Leavitt JW. Typhoid Mary: Captive to the Public's Health. Boston: Beacon Press, 1996.

[21] Clayton EW, Steinberg KK, Khoury MJ, *et al.* Informed consent for genetic research in stored tissue samples. JAMA 1995;274:1786-92.

[22] Hunter D, Caporaso N. Informed consent in epidemiologic studies involving genetic markers. Epidemiology 1997;8:596-9.

[23] American Society for Human Genetics. ASHG report: statement on informed consent for genetic research. Am J Hum Genet 1996;59:471-4.

[24] Andrews L, Nelkin D. Whose body is it anyway? Disputes over body tissue in a biotechnology age. Lancet 1998;351:53.

[25] Oppenheimer GM. In the eye of the storm: the epidemiological construction of AIDS. In: Fee E, Fox DM, Eds. AIDS: The Burdens of History. Berkeley: University of California Press, 1988; pp. 267-300.

[26] Farmer P. AIDS and acusation: Haiti and the Geography of Blame. Berkeley: University of California Press, 1992.

[27] Gold EB. Confidentiality and privacy protection in epidemiologic research. In: Coughlin SS, Beauchamp TL, Eds. Ethics and Epidemiology: New York: Oxford University Press, 1996; pp. 128-41.

[28] Gostin LO, Lazzarini Z, Neslund VS, Osterholm MT. The public health information infrastructure: a national review of the law on health information privacy. JAMA 1996;275:1921-7.

[29] Noble EP. The DRD2 gene, smoking, and lung cancer (editorial). J Natl Cancer Inst 1998;90:343-5.

[30] Keet IP, Klein MR, Just JJ, *et al.* The role of host genetics in the natural history of HIV-1 infection: the needle in the haystack. AIDS 1996;10(Suppl A):559-67.

[31]   Andrews LB, Fullarton JE, Holtzman NA, Motulsky AG, Eds. Assessing Genetic Risks: Implications for Health and Social Policy. Washington, DC: Institute of Medicine, 1994.

[32]   Annas GJ, Elias S. Gene Mapping: Using Law and Ethics as Guides. New York: Oxford University Press, 1992.

[33]   Engelhardt HT, Jr, Caplan AL, Eds. Scientific Controversies: Case Studies in the Resolution and Closure of Disputes in Science and Technology. New York: Cambridge University Press, 1987.

[34]   Bronowski J. Science and Human Values. New York: Harper & Row, 1956.

[35]   Proctor RN. Cancer Wars: How Politics Shapes What We Know and Don't Know about Cancer. New York: Basic Books, 1995.

[36]   Weed DL. Undetermination and incommensurability in contemporary epidemiology. Kennedy Inst Ethics J 1997;7:107-27.

[37]   Rothman KJ, Cann CI. Judging words rather than authors (editorial). Epidemiology 1987;8:223-5.

CHAPTER 5

Emerging Paradigms in Epidemiology and Public Health: Metaphors and Conceptual Models

Abstract. Metaphors and visual images have been used in epidemiology in conjunction with frameworks and theories proposed to explain disease causation and the processes that give rise to social patterning of disease risks and the ways in which risk behaviors arise and become maintained in social groups. The metaphor of a running stream has recently been extended by Glass and McAttee to stimulate creative thinking about the determinants of risk behaviors in populations and emerging paradigms of disease causation. The frameworks and theories that have been proposed to illustrate or explain the processes that give rise to social patterning of disease have been paralleled by the development and refinement of methods of multilevel statistical analysis and complex systems modeling in public health. The metaphors and conceptual models employed in epidemiology have moved beyond short, causal chains and reductionist world-views to include more holistic, dynamic perspectives that are more consistent with the complexity of real world situations.

INTRODUCTION

Epidemiologists and other public health researchers have seen a range of metaphors used in conjunction with conceptual models and theories of disease causation. An early example is the metaphor of a "web of causation" which implies that effects such as disease outcomes do not depend on single, isolated causes, but rather occur as the result of complex chains of causation in which each link has many antecedents [1, 2]. More recently, the "Chinese boxes" metaphor was used by Susser and Susser to illustrate their eco-epidemiology paradigm which encompasses many levels of organization including molecular, individual, and societal [3]. The hierarchical or multilevel structure of this model of disease causation extends from individual-level biological or nonbiological risk factors to more distal societal factors [3]. A further example is the "fractal metaphor" employed by Kreiger in conjunction with ecosocial theory [4, 5]. The fractal metaphor invites consideration of the conjoint expression of biological and social factors at different levels, from the molecular biology of cells to population rates of disease, and also takes into account a population's history, culture, and socioeconomic relationships [5]. The eco-epidemiology paradigm proposed by Susser and Susser [3] and the ecosocial theory discussed by Kreiger [4, 5] offer greater insights into disease determinants at the individual versus population level compared with early metaphors such as the "web of causation" and "causal chain." For many important public health

Steven S. Coughlin

problems (for example, traumatic injuries and major depression [6, 7], these metaphors and ecosocial models of disease causation may help to clarify useful areas for further research or point to possible avenues for public health interventions.

Metaphors and visual images have also been used in conjunction with frameworks and theories proposed to explain the processes that give rise to social patterning of disease risks and the ways in which risk behaviors arise and become maintained in social groups [5, 8]. The stream metaphor did not arise in public health but can rather be traced back over a hundred years to psychological and philosophical traditions such as William James' theory of mind [9]. In the public health literature, the metaphor of a "running stream" has been used to describe the chain of causal influences that extends from proximate, individual factors to more distal social factors [8, 10, 11]. Glass and McAtee modified and enhanced the metaphor of a running stream by extending it along two axes. In their account, time is represented on one axis (for example, the life course from conception to death) and levels of biological or social organization or nested systems are represented on the other axis [8]. The framework integrates biological factors such as genes, cells, and organs and socioenvironmental influences on health behaviors. The nested systems included in the framework extend from genes, to cells and organs, to social networks, groups, culture, and the global environment. According to this metaphorical representation of the multileveled processes that create population patterns of health, people "are like buoyant objects floating in a network of tributaries, streams, and rivers" [8]. The metaphor also asserts that "The watershed might contain bumps, hills, or mountains that parallel barriers to adoption of health promoting behaviors." Social structures (for example, urban sprawl, and opportunities for exercise or maintaining a healthy diet, and other changes in the physical environment that may be related to the obesity epidemic) are represented in Glass and McAtee's metaphor as rocks, boulders, valleys, canyons, hills, and man-made structures such as river channels that shape and constrain the flow of water over time (where water represents health-related behaviors such as physical activity and diet) [8]. The framework proposed by Glass and McAtee, which can be tied to earlier multilevel paradigms such as eco-epidemiology and concepts of life-course epidemiology,[3, 12, 13] may be useful for generating theories of disease causation and for thinking about social and biological influences of behaviors and disease. For example, the framework suggests that uphill forces (e.g., government policies) may have greater leverage in shaping the flow of health behaviors than factors that exert their influence at the level of social networks.

There are notable differences between Glass and McAtee's framework for accounting for the determinants of risk behaviors in populations and previous paradigms of disease causation such as the "eco-epidemiology" paradigm proposed by Susser and Susser [3]. For example, time is a separate axis in Glass and McAtee's framework but not in the eco-epidemiology framework. A more striking departure from previous frameworks is that Glass and McAtee do not argue that social conditions (for example, income inequity, discrimination, population density, or neighborhood social disorganization) are causes of disease in the traditional epidemiologic sense. Rather, they view social conditions as *risk regulators* that influence behavioral risk in ways that are nonspecific, subject to temporal variation, and contingent upon intermediate processes [8]. According to Glass and McAtee there is a need to identify potentially powerful "levers of behavior change at the population level" (for example, laws, policies, and regulations, neighborhood and community conditions, and behavioral norms, rules, and expectations) even if those factors cannot meet "demanding epistemological criteria for causation." [8]. In their account, risk regulators are relatively stable features of social and physical environments "that impose constraints and opportunities that shape, channel, motivate and induce behavioral risk factors that cause disease, and the salutary factors that protect against exposure and delay disease progression." [8]. Seen from this perspective, risk regulators are not risk factors *per se* but rather social conditions that regulate or influence probabilities of exposure to behaviors that lead to illness.

The framework provided by Glass and McAtee does have certain desirable features, for example, its suitability for describing or stimulating creative thinking about causal influences related to behavioral risk factors at the micro-level (groups, family, social networks), mezzo-level (work-sites, schools, communities, and healthcare facilities), macro-level (national, state, and large-area dynamics), and global-level (geopolitical, economic, and environmental dynamics) [8]. However, the framework also has certain disadvantages including its focus on risk of disease onset and disease progression and apparent neglect of other outcomes (for example, disease morbidity, disability, quality of life, and mortality). A further issue is that the framework provided by Glass and McAtee may be more suitable for describing the causal influences that account for adult-onset chronic diseases (for example, obesity and coronary heart disease) than those that account for some other health problems. Another disadvantage may be that risk regulators, as defined by Glass and McAtee, are not necessarily causally related to the outcomes of interest. Rather, risk regulators operate through multiple pathways and up- or down-regulate the likelihood of key risk factors (for example, physical inactivity, a poor diet, or cigarette smoking) [8]. If risk regulators are not causally related to the outcomes of interest, then it is not clear how modifying such risk regulators would provide "leverage" to increase healthy behaviors or reduce illness at the population level. The framework provided by Glass and McAtee does not provide clear guidance of how to determine which risk regulators should be modified in order to improve population health. This leaves open the possibility that risk regulators might be targeted that have little or no impact on risk behaviors or population health or that have unexpected side effects. For example, efforts to decrease population density or improve the desirability of neighborhoods might decrease the amount of affordable housing or require some low-income residents to commute long distances to get to work. Of course, a variety of legal and social arguments can be advanced to counter such social problems as discrimination and neighborhood social disorganization even if the evidence for a causal relationship with some health outcomes may be difficult to confirm in public health studies.

The frameworks and theories have been proposed to illustrate or explain the processes that give rise to social patterning of disease risks (for example, ecological models of disease causation) have been paralleled by the development and refinement of advanced methods of statistical analysis and modeling. One notable example is multilevel statistical models which have been widely used in epidemiologic and public health research [14, 15]. As noted by Diez Roux [14], multilevel analysis allows researchers to move beyond theory and speculation and empirically test specific aspects of theoretical models having to do with multilevel determinants of health. McMichael and others have called for the use of multilevel or pathway modeling in epidemiology, pointing out that by using such statistical models and collaborating with other disciplines, epidemiologists could develop quantitative and structural analyses of how social variables affect health outcomes [16]. Multilevel analysis enables researchers to analyze data using statistical approaches that are more compatible with socioecological frameworks for understanding determinants of health in populations. Effects of group-level characteristics (for example, characteristics of neighborhoods) have been observed across a wide range of health outcomes, independent of individual-level factors. The advantages of multilevel statistical techniques include their flexibility and generality and the ability to test for interactions between individual-level and contextual factors, although multilevel analyses do have certain shortcomings [15]. One limitation is that multilevel models do not take into account feedback loops [14]. Another limitation is that many multilevel analyses have been cross-sectional in nature rather than analyses of longitudinal data. Cross-sectional studies may have limited ability to decipher temporal relationships between some individual- or group-level variables and the outcome of interest. A further issue is that published studies have been inconsistent in controlling for individual-level variables. There may be uncertainty about whether individual-level variables should be conceptualized as confounders, mediators, or modifiers of the effect of the associations between group-level variables and the outcome of interest [17]. In some studies, questions have been raised over model misspecification resulting from omitted or mismeasured individual- and group-level variables. In order to address such concerns, investigators should consider employing a conceptual framework or logic model that clarifies the pathways by which various individual- and group-level variables, alone or in combination, are associated with the outcome of interest. Once such framework is a directed acyclic graph.

Another development that has paralleled the emergence of new frameworks and theories to explain the social patterning of disease risks is complex systems modeling in public health (for example, dynamic systems modeling). The paradigm or perspective that underlies complex systems modeling considers the connections among different components, including feedback loops and changes over time, and thus is well-suited to address the dynamic complexity of many public health issues [18, 19]. Dynamic systems modeling involves the development of computer simulation models that may be tested systematically to find optimal policies in public health, healthcare, and other fields. Horner and Hirsch observed that "System dynamics shows promise as a means of modeling multiple interacting diseases and risks, the interaction of delivery systems and disease populations, and matters of national and state policy" [19]. What are needed are analytic methods that can address situations of dynamic complexity in which the needs of populations and groups change over time and in which risk factors, diseases, and healthcare resources are in a state of continuous interaction and flux [19]. System dynamics modeling entails the development of causal diagrams and computer simulation models that allow for alternative policies and scenarios to be tested in a systematic way [20].

To cite one example, there has been extensive discussion and debate over how best to identify and treat mild traumatic brain injury among returning combat veterans and other populations, especially in situations where brain injury may overlap with posttraumatic stress disorder (PTSD) [21-24]. A systems perspective supports the view that there are likely many opportunities to intervene to assist persons with traumatic brain injury (for example, through the development of improved screening and diagnostic tools, multidisciplinary health care teams and integrated systems of care, amelioration of current or persisting symptoms and co-morbid conditions, family support, public and professional education, and provision of job training, educational, and rehabilitative services). And, that the need for each of these components is likely to change or evolve over time, at the population or group level, as in a dynamic system. Dynamic systems modeling, especially if combined with longitudinal epidemiologic and clinical studies and health services research, might be helpful for identifying high leverage intervention points or refined policies. As this example suggests, complex systems modeling is likely to be a useful tool to plan and evaluate health interventions to address important public health concerns such as traumatic brain injury and PTSD. Related tools and techniques—those of operational systems engineering—have recently been discussed in relation to the quality of the U.S. Department of Defense military health care delivery system, including how to improve the tracking and navigation of patients with severe traumatic brain injury through critical transition points (for example, transitions from a health care organization in one military service to a facility in another, or to a Department of Veterans Affairs or civilian health care facility) [25].

In summary, several metaphors have been used in epidemiology and public health, in conjunction with conceptual models and theories of disease causation, including the web of causation, the Chinese boxes metaphor, the fractal metaphor, and the running stream metaphor conjoined with systems thinking. The metaphor of a running stream has recently been extended by Glass and McAttee to stimulate creative thinking about the determinants of risk behaviors in populations and emerging paradigms of disease causation [8]. The emergence of new frameworks and theories to explain the social patterning of disease risks has been paralleled by the development of refined methods of multilevel statistical analysis and complex systems modeling in public health (for example, systems engineering and dynamic systems modeling). The metaphors and conceptual models employed in epidemiology have moved beyond short, causal chains and reductionist world-views to include more holistic, dynamic perspectives that are more consistent with the complexity of real world situations. As noted by Leischow and Milstein [18], systems thinking often changes our perception of what the problems are, where their boundaries lie, and how we should approach them.

REFERENCES

[1]   MacMahon B, Pugh TF, *et al*. Epidemiologic Methods. Boxton: Little, Brown and Company, 1960.

[2]   Mausner JS, Bahn AK. Epidemiology. An Introductory Text. Philadelphia: W.B.

Saunders Company, 1974.

[3]   Susser M, Susser E. Choosing a future for epidemiology: II. From black box to Chinese Boxes and eco-epidemiology. Am J Public Health 1996;86:674-7.

[4]   Krieger N. Epidemiology and the web of causation: has anyone seen the spider? Soc Sci Med 1994;39:887-903.

[5]   Krieger N. Sticky webs, hungry spiders, buzzing flies, and fractal metaphors: on the misleading juxtaposition of "risk factor" versus "social" epidemiology (editorial). J Epidemiol Commun Health 1999;53:678-80.

[6]   Summers CR, Ivins B, Schwab KA. Traumatic brain injury in the United States: an epidemiologic overview. Mt Sinai J Med 2009;76:105-10.

[7]   Calhoun PS, Wiley M, Dennis MF, Beckham JC. Self-reported health and physician diagnosed illnesses in women with posttraumatic stress disorder and major depressive disorder. J Trauma Stress 2009;22:122-30.

[8]   Glass TA, McAttee MJ. Behavioral science at the crossroads in public health: extending horizons, envisioning the future. Soc Sci Med 2006;62:1650-71.

[9]   Gruber HE, Bodeker K, Eds. Creativity, Psychology and the History of Science. Dordrect, The Netherlands: Springer, 2005.

[10]   Anonymous. Population health looking upstream (editorial). Lancet 1994;343:429-30.

[11]   Kaplan GA. Where do shared pathways lead? Some reflections on a research agenda. Psychosom Med 1995;57:208-12.

[12]   Coughlin SS. Scientific paradigms in epidemiology and professional values (commentary). Epidemiology 1998;9:578-80.

[13]   Davey Smith G, Ed. Health Inequalities: Lifecourse Approaches. Bristol, United Kingdom: The Policy Press, 2003.

[14]   Diez Roux AV. Next steps in understanding the multilevel determinants of health. J Epidemiol Commun Health 2008;62:957-9.

[15]   Coughlin SS. Multilevel analysis in health services research (editorial). Open Health Serv Policy J 2009;2:42-44.

[16]   McMichael AJ. Prisoners of the proximate: loosening the constraints on epidemiology in an age of change. Am J Epidemiol 1999;149:887-97.

[17]   Riva M, Gauvin L, Barnett TA. Toward the next generation of research into small area effects on health: a synthesis of multilevel investigations published since July 1998. J Epidemiol Comm Health 2007;61:853-61.

[18]   Leischow SJ, Milstein B. Systems thinking and modeling for public health practice. Am J Public Health 2006;96:403-5

[19]   Hormer JB, Hirsch GB. System dynamics modeling for public health: background and opportunities. Am J Public Health 2006;96:452-8.

[20]   Sterman JD. Learning from evidence in a complex world. Am J Public Health 2006;96:505-14.

[21]   Belanger HG, Oomoto JM, Vanderploeg RD. The Veterans health Administration system of Care for mild traumatic brain injury: costs, benefits, and controversies. J Health Trauma Rehabil 2009;24:4-13.

[22]   Hill JJ III, Mobo BHP Jr., Cullen MR. Separating deployment-related traumatic brain injury and posttraumatic stress disorder in veterans. Preliminary findings from the Veterans Affairs Traumatic Brain Injury Screening Program. Am J Phys Med Rehabil 2009;88:605-14.

[23]   Bryant RA. Disentangling mild traumatic brain injury and stress reactions. N Engl J Med 2008;358:525-7.

[24]   Hoge CW, Goldberg HM, Castro CA. Care of war veterans with mild traumatic brain injury—flawed perspectives (commentary). N Engl J Med 2009;360:1588-91.

[25]   Butler D, Buono J, Erdtmann F, Reid P, Eds. Systems Engineering to Improve Traumatic Brain Injury Care in the Military Health System. National Academy of Engineering and Institute of Medicine. Washington, DC: National Academies Press, 2008.

CHAPTER 6

Genetic Variants and Individual- and Societal-Level Factors

Abstract. Over the past decade, leading epidemiologists have noted the importance of social factors in studying and understanding the distribution and determinants of disease in human populations; but to what extent are epidemiologic studies integrating genetic information and other biologic variables with information about individual-level risk factors and group-level or societal factors related to the broader residential, behavioral, or cultural context? There remains a need to consider ways to integrate genetic information with social and contextual information in epidemiologic studies, partly to combat the overemphasis on the importance of genetic factors as determinants of disease in human populations. Even in genome-wide association studies of coronary heart disease and other common complex diseases, only a small proportion of heritability is explained by the genetic variants identified to date. It is possible that familial clustering due to genetic factors has been overestimated and that important environmental or social influences (acting alone or in combination with genetic variants) have been overlooked.

INTRODUCTION

Over the past decade, several authors have called for new research paradigms in epidemiology that more adequately take into account different levels of analysis at the molecular, individual, and societal or group levels [1, 2]. For example, in a far-ranging commentary published in the *American Journal of Epidemiology* in 1998, Diez-Roux (1) noted the resurgence of interest in the social origins of disease, echoing observations made by other epidemiologists about the importance of social factors in studying and understanding the distribution and determinants of disease in human populations [2-5]. Diez-Roux noted that epidemiology may be on the brink of a new genetic paradigm, and pointed to the development of new genetic technologies and the explosive growth in research on the genetics and molecular mechanisms of disease [1]. However, the major thrust of her commentary was to underscore the importance of assessing both population risk factors for disease that exist at the group level (e.g., neighborhood effects) and more proximal risk factors that exist at the individual level (e.g., biological variables or genetic traits assessed using the methods of molecular genetics). This approach allows biologic phenomena to be viewed within their social contexts and for individual-level explanations of disease causation to be integrated into broader models that incorporate interactions between individuals as well as group-level determinants and effect modifiers [1]. The

Steven S. Coughlin

approach outlined by Diez-Roux is consistent with the eco-epidemiology paradigm proposed by Susser and Susser [2] which encompasses many levels of organization including molecular, individual, and societal. The hierarchical or multilevel structure of this model of disease causation extends from individual-level biologic or nonbiologic risk factors to more distal societal factors. From this perspective, incorporating information about the societal determinants of disease is key since the model may overemphasize the importance of more proximal factors at the individual level if group-level or societal determinants of health are ignored [1].

In view of the calls by Diez-Roux, Susser and Susser, and others, more than a decade ago, for a new paradigm for epidemiologic research, it is worthwhile to consider the extent to which epidemiologic studies are integrating genetic information (and other biologic variables) with information about individual-level risk factors and group-level or societal factors related to the broader residential, behavioral, or cultural context. A recent commentary by Khoury and Wacholder [6], who defined "environment" broadly, noted that the proportion of articles reporting on gene-environment interactions remains at about 14% in the total Human Genome Epidemiology Network literature. However, the proportion of articles that examined effect modification by group-level or societal determinants of health is likely to have been much smaller than 14%.

Bressler *et al.* [7] recently reported that two of the genetic variants previously identified by Wellcome Trust Case Control Consortium case-control studies (rs1333049 and rs501120) were independently associated with incident coronary heart disease (CHD) among white participants in the Atherosclerosis Risk in Communities Study, even after adjustment for multiple established risk factors for CHD. The established CHD risk factors adjusted for by Bressler *et al.* [7] consisted of age, body mass index (BMI), high density lipoprotein (HDL) cholesterol, low density lipoprotein (LDL) cholesterol, diabetes, hypertension, and smoking. Other established risk factors for CHD (e.g., physical inactivity) and nontraditional or emerging risk factors such as pro-thrombotic factors were not controlled for in the analysis. Physical activity has been inversely associated with CHD in several epidemiologic studies after adjustment for other CHD risk factors [8]. Possible pathways for a beneficial effect of exercise on CHD risk include the lowering of blood pressure and improvement of body composition, glucose tolerance, HDL cholesterol function, or thrombotic function [8]. The relationship between a sport activity index and CHD risk has previously been examined among participants in the Atherosclerosis Risk in Communities Study [9].

The decisions made by Bressler *et al.* about which CHD risk factors to adjust for in the analysis are important partly because they considered a two-sided P value of < 0.05 to be statistically significant and the magnitudes of the observed associations were quite modest. The observed P value for rs501120 was 0.01 and the point estimate of the hazard rate ratio was only 1.18 (95% confidence interval 1.05, 1.33) after adjustment for age, gender, BMI, smoking, diabetes, hypertension, HDL cholesterol, and LDL cholesterol [7]. It would be helpful to have more information about why the authors preferred to use this particular set of risk factors for CHD and what procedures they followed to identify potentially confounding variables and effect modifiers, either at the individual level or the group level. Perhaps their findings might have been different if they had also adjusted for physical activity, socioeconomic status, alcohol consumption, or factors associated with thrombotic function. Of course, the pathways by which CHD risk factors exert their effects on CHD risk at the individual-level (e.g., physical activity) or group-level (for example, neighborhood characteristics linked to alcohol consumption, diet, cigarette smoking, and obesity) may involve factors already addressed in the study by Bressler *et al.* such as HDL and LDL cholesterol or hypertension.

One of the issues raised by Bressler *et al.* is how to distinguish between "established" and "non-established" risk factors for CHD? Some frequently cited risk factors for CHD (e.g., obesity and body shape or waist-to-hip ratio) have been considered established risk factors by some authors but not others. Thus, in the context of evolving scientific information and diversity of opinions about what constitutes an established risk factor for common complex diseases such as CHD it is likely to be important for researchers conducting molecular epidemiology studies to go beyond adjusting for a minimum set of traditional risk factors and to more thoroughly explore potential confounding and effect modification by several traditional and nontraditional risk factors.

What about the need to control for group-level variables such as neighborhood effects, or to consider the possibility of effect modification by group-level variables? Should group-level variables be routinely incorporated into molecular epidemiology research such as the study by Bressler *et al.*? Although studies have demonstrated that group-level variables such as neighborhood characteristics influence CHD risk factors such as cigarette smoking, obesity, and socioeconomic status [10, 11], investigators studying group-level factors associated with CHD risk often test specific hypotheses and consider how neighborhood effects may be mediated through traditional CHD risk factors. In addition, the number of group-level variables that could be assessed in any given study (given sufficient time and resources) is very large. Testing for effect modification by a large number of group-level variables could result in some interaction terms being found to be statistically significant by chance alone especially in studies involving large numbers of research participants. Thus, it is not clear that epidemiologists should routinely assess uncontrolled confounding or effect modification by group-level variables in studies that examine associations with individual-level variables including genetic variants and other biologic factors.

Nevertheless, molecular epidemiology studies that do assess interactions with group-level variables may be informative such as when they are designed to test specific hypotheses about possible causal pathways. Thus, there remains a need to consider ways to integrate genetic information with social and contextual information in epidemiologic studies, partly to combat the overemphasis of the importance of genetic factors as determinants of disease in human populations. As Ioannidis *et al.* [12, p. 2] noted, "There is a special enthusiasm about the potential power of genomics to define the etiology of disease and phenotypes..." There may be a tendency to view associations with genetic factors as causal and associations with factors related to the broader social, cultural, or behavioral context as noncausal. Genetic and biologic factors are commonly considered to be foundational in hierarchical models and theories of disease causation, even though, as Parascandola and Weed [13] noted, there is no reason to assume that causes at the genetic or molecular level are any more "real" or significant than causes as another level such as social factors. Even in genome-wide association studies of CHD and other common complex diseases, only a small proportion of heritability is explained by the genetic variants identified to date [14]. It is possible that familial clustering due to genetic factors has been overestimated and that important environmental or social influences (acting alone or in combination with genetic variants) have been overlooked. There may be a tendency to inadequately take into account the complexity of the human biological, physical, and social environment, or the potential for confounding or effect modification by unmeasured genetic or environmental factors.

A particular challenge is the current lack of information about mechanisms of disease at the molecular, cellular, individual, and societal levels. Although an increasing number of genetic markers are being identified for CHD and many other diseases and health conditions, important questions remain to be answered about biologic and physiologic processes that may account for replicable associations with genetic markers. Genetic markers such as those examined in genome-wide association studies and some molecular epidemiology studies may be far removed from complex physiologic processes that are more important risk factors for disease [6]. In addition, individual-level and societal-level risk factors, examined in other epidemiologic studies, may represent only crude markers of disease risk and not provide detailed information about causal pathways.

In conclusion, although there has been increasing recognition of the desirability of not conceptualizing determinants of disease solely in terms of molecular or biologic factors and striving to also conceptualize them in terms of the broader social, cultural, or behavioral context, not all epidemiologic studies include or should include group-level or societal-level factors. For studies that do include such variables, investigators should consider developing a conceptual framework (i.e., a logic model) that clarifies the pathways by which various individual- or group-level variables, alone or in combination, are associated with the outcome of interest [3, 5].

REFERENCES

[1]   Diez-Roux AV. On genes, individuals, society, and epidemiology. Am J Epidemiol 1998;148:1027-32.

[2]   Susser M, Susser E. Choosing a future for epidemiology: II. From black box to Chinese Boxes and eco-epidemiology. Am J Public Health 1996;86:674-7.

[3]   McMichael AJ. Prisoners of the proximate: loosening the constraints on epidemiology in an age of change. Am J Epidemiol 1999;149:887-97.

[4]   Pearce N. Traditional epidemiology, modern epidemiology, and public health. Am J Public Health 1996;86:678-83.

[5]   Krieger N. Epidemiology and the web of causation: has anyone seen the spider? Soc Sci Med 1994;39:887-903.

[6]   Khoury MJ, Wacholder S. Invited commentary: from genome-wide association studies to gene-environment-wide interaction studies—challenges and opportunities. Am J Epidemiol 2008;169:227-30.

[7]   Bressler J, Folsom AR, Couper DJ, *et al.* Genetic variants identified in a European genome-wide association study that were found to predict incident coronary heart disease in the Atherosclerosis Risk in Communities Study. Am J Epidemiol 2010;171:14-23.

[8]   Sesso HD, Paffenbarger RS, Jr, Lee I-M. Physical activity and coronary heart disease in men. The Harvard Alumni Health Study. Circulation 2000;102:975-

80.

[9]   Chambless LE, Folsom AR, Sharrett AR, *et al*. Coronary heart disease risk prediction in the Atherosclerosis Risk in Communities (ARIC) Study. J Clin Epidemiol 2003;56:880-90.

[10]   Moore LV, Diez Roux AV, Nettleton JA, *et al*. Fast-food consumption, diet quality, and neighborhood exposure to fast food. The Multi-Ethnic Study of Atherosclerosis. Am J Epidemiol 2009;170:29-36.

[11]   Diez Roux AV, Stein Merkin S, Arnett D, *et al*. Neighborhood of residence and incidence of coronary heart disease. N Engl J Med 2001;345:99-106.

[12]   Ioannidis JPA, Boffetta P, Little J, *et al*. Assessment of cumulative evidence on genetic associations: interim guidelines. Int J Epidemiol 2007;1-11.

[13]   Parascandola M, Weed DL. Causation in epidemiology. J Epidemiol Community Health 2001;55:905-12.

[14]   Pearson TA, Manolio TA. How to interpret a genome-wide association study. JAMA 2008;299:1335-44.

CHAPTER 7

Research Paradigms and the Strengthening of Causal Inference in Epidemiology

Abstract: Changes in research paradigms and theories about disease causation have frequently led to refinements in frameworks for causal inference. Among the most promising paradigm shifts in contemporary epidemiology has been an increasing willingness to examine disease etiology using a multilevel or systems approach and a parallel trend towards the mathematization of causal inference. However, these two important developments (adoption of a multilevel or systems approach for epidemiologic research and use of quantitative models for causal inference) have not been adequately linked. One important impediment to reaching the full potential of multilevel studies is the need for further refinement of quantitative and graphical models for causal inference that are suitable for emerging research paradigms. More efforts should be made to clarify conceptually what approaches work best for identifying causal relationships in the context of complex systems. Optimal approaches to causal inference are not necessarily identical across epidemiology subdisciplines and researchers should not assume that there is one correct or optimal theory of causality that accounts for causal relationships identified in epidemiologic research.

INTRODUCTION

Among scholars from different disciplines and professions–including epidemiologists and philosophers of science–there is a natural tendency to discuss causal inference in the context of particular research paradigms. Thus, it should come as no surprise that the sizeable literature on causal inference in epidemiologic research frequently mentions historical shifts in paradigms for epidemiologic and public health research. Examples include the shift from the miasma theory of disease causation to the germ theory in the nineteenth century and the transition that occurred in the twentieth century from a focus on infectious diseases linked to particular organisms to a focus on chronic conditions such as cancer and cardiovascular disease that have a multifactorial etiology [1, 2]. Indeed, changes in research paradigms and theories about disease causation have frequently led to refinements in frameworks for causal inference. More recent examples can also be cited. For example, technological advances in molecular epidemiology and human genome research have led to proposals for refined methods for assessing associations in genome-wide association studies [3]. Among the most promising paradigm shifts in contemporary epidemiology, however, have been an increasing willingness to examine disease etiology using a multilevel or systems approach and a parallel trend towards the mathematization of causal inference [4-13]. However, these two important developments (adoption of a multilevel or systems approach for epidemiologic research and use of quantitative models for causal inference) have not been adequately linked.

In this concluding chapter, I argue several inter-related points. The first is that emerging paradigms in epidemiologic research that take into account different levels of organization (for example, molecular, individual, and societal) can help to strengthen causal inference in observational research. The second is that several impediments remain to be addressed before the full potential of such multilevel studies can be realized. These impediments include the need for further refinement of quantitative models for causal inference that are suitable for emerging research paradigms. The final point argued below is that optimal approaches to causal inference are not necessarily identical across epidemiology subdisciplines such as genetic epidemiology and social epidemiology. Moreover, researchers should not assume that there is one correct or optimal theory of causality that accounts for causal relationships identified in epidemiologic research. I will address each one of these points in turn.

THE SYSTEMS APPROACH AND HOW IT CAN HELP TO STRENGTHEN CAUSAL INFERENCE IN EPIDEMIOLOGY

Systems thinking and the relationships between systems analysis and causal inference have been increasingly addressed in the epidemiology literature [10, 14-16]. As discussed earlier in this volume, Susser and Susser called for a paradigm shift from the emphasis on individual risk factors for disease to a new ecologic approach (a "Chinese boxes paradigm" or "eco-epidemiology"), which encompasses many levels of organization, including molecular, individual, and societal [14]. The hierarchical or multilevel structure of this model of disease causation extends from individual-level biological or nonbiological risk factors to more distal societal factors. Similarly, the ecosocial theory outlined by Kreiger [15] entails the conjoint expression of biological and social factors at different levels, from the molecular biology of cells to population rates of disease, and also takes into account a population's history, culture, and socioeconomic relationships. These frameworks for disease causation are helping to clarify useful areas for further research for many important public health problems. The framework proposed by Glass and McAtee [16] may also be useful for generating theories of disease causation and for thinking about social and biological influences of behaviors and disease. The framework integrates biological factors such as genes, cells, and organs and socioenvironmental influences on health behaviors. The nested systems included in the framework extend from genes, cells, and organs, to social networks, groups, culture, and the global environment.

The framework proposed by Glass and McAtee, which is closely related to multilevel paradigms such as eco-epidemiology and concepts of life-course epidemiology, provides a useful example for thinking about the challenges of causal inference in complex systems [16]. According to Glass and McAtee there is a need to identify potential levers of behavior change at the population level (for example, laws, policies, and regulations, neighborhood and community conditions, and behavioral norms, rules, and expectations) even if those factors cannot meet demanding criteria for causation. However, Glass and McAtee do not argue that social conditions are causes of disease in the traditional epidemiologic sense. Rather, they view social conditions as *risk regulators* that influence behavioral risk in ways that are nonspecific, subject to temporal variation, and contingent upon intermediate processes [16]. In their account, risk regulators regulate or influence probabilities of exposure to behaviors that lead to illness. If risk regulators are not causally related to the outcomes of interest, then it is not clear how modifying such risk regulators would provide "leverage" to increase healthy behaviors or reduce illness at the population level. The framework provided by Glass and McAtee does not provide clear guidance of how to determine which risk regulators should be modified in order to improve population health. This leaves open the possibility that risk regulators might be targeted that have little or no impact on risk behaviors or population health or that have unexpected side effects.

The frameworks and theories that have been proposed to illustrate or explain the processes that give rise to social patterning of diseases have been paralleled by the development and refinement of improved methods of statistical analysis and modeling. One notable example is multilevel statistical models which have been widely used in epidemiologic and public health research. As noted by Diez Roux [11], multilevel analysis allows researchers to move beyond theory and speculation and empirically test specific aspects of theoretical models having to do with multilevel determinants of health. Several authors have called for the use of multilevel analysis in epidemiology, pointing out that by using such statistical models and collaborating with other disciplines, epidemiologists could develop quantitative and structural analyses of how social variables affect health outcomes [10-12, 14, 15]. Multilevel analysis enables researchers to analyze data using statistical approaches that are more compatible with socioecological frameworks for understanding determinants of health in populations. Effects of group-level characteristics (for example, characteristics of neighborhoods) have been observed across a wide range of health outcomes, independent of individual-level factors [11]. The advantages of multilevel statistical techniques include their flexibility and generality and the ability to test for interactions between individual-level and contextual factors, although multilevel analyses do have certain shortcomings. One limitation is that multilevel models do not take into account feedback loops [11]. Another limitation is that many multilevel analyses have been cross-sectional in nature rather than analyses of longitudinal data [12]. Cross-sectional studies may have limited ability to decipher temporal relationships between some individual- or group-level variables and the outcome of interest. A further issue is that published studies have been inconsistent in controlling for individual-level variables. There may be uncertainty about whether individual-level variables should be conceptualized as confounders, mediators, or modifiers of the effect of the associations between group-level variables and the outcome of interest [11, 17]. In some studies, questions have been raised over model misspecification resulting from omitted or mismeasured individual- and group-level variables. In order to address such concerns, investigators should employ a conceptual framework or logic model to clarify the pathways by which various individual- and group-level variables, alone or in combination, are associated with the outcome of interest.

Despite the utility of multilevel statistical analysis for analyzing data from ecological studies and other epidemiologic studies influenced by emerging research paradigms, the probabilistic relationships identified through such analyses are likely to represent only surface phenomena of underlying causal mechanisms and relationships [6]. There are several remaining impediments to clarifying causal relationships as discussed below.

IMPEDIMENTS TO REACHING THE FULL POTENTIAL OF MULTILEVEL STUDIES TO CLARIFY CAUSAL RELATIONSHIPS

One important impediment to reaching the full potential of multilevel studies to clarify causal relationships is the need for further refinement of quantitative and graphical models for causal inference that are suitable for emerging research paradigms. Although several authors have clarified the relevance of counterfactual models to epidemiologic research [5, 8, 9, 18], more work needs to be done to apply counterfactual concepts and methods to ecological frameworks for disease causation and systems analysis. There has been some discussion of applications of the counterfactual causal framework to multilevel health research [18, 19] but more work in this area is needed. In the literature on causal inference in social epidemiology, there has sometimes been a tendency to focus on questions pertaining to what constitutes a causal factor (for example, whether immutable factors such as age and race should be considered causal factors) and to avoid delving deeply into the equally important topic of how best to warrant causal relationships in social epidemiologic studies. Recent articles by Oakes [19] and others have helped to fill this gap. In many contemporary areas of research, complex causation and systems thinking are of interest, but there is lingering concern that some associations identified through complex systems modeling and other innovative approaches may not be causal in the traditional epidemiologic sense. Thus, more concerted efforts should be made to clarify conceptually what approaches work best for identifying causal relationships in the context of complex systems.

One area ripe for further methodological research is the use of structural equations and graphical models to help clarify causal and non-causal associations in epidemiologic studies [20-22]. Directed acyclic graphs, which figure prominently in Bayes-net methods [6, 23], have been discussed in relation to measurement bias in epidemiologic studies [22]. However, to date, there has been no comprehensive effort to apply such methods to the analysis of data from multilevel studies that encompass many levels of organization (for example, molecular, individual, and societal). Both ecological and individual-level variables included in multilevel analyses are subject to differential or nondifferential measurement error. Causal diagrams can be used to represent biases that arise from confounding, selection, and measurement [22].

WHY OPTIMAL APPROACHES TO CAUSAL INFERENCE ARE NOT NECESSARILY IDENTICAL ACROSS EPIDEMIOLOGY SUBDISCIPLINES

As noted by Carthwright [23], a well-known philosopher of science, we are used to thinking of causation as one thing, even though we may accept that there are different methods to learn about it. This is true in epidemiology where we are used to thinking about causal inference as a monolithic concept that cuts across epidemiologic subdisciplines. However, there are increasing indications that this is a mistake. For example, the causal models and frameworks that apply to molecular epidemiology and genetics are not necessarily the same as those that apply to infectious disease epidemiology or to the complex social and economic systems that are of interest in social epidemiology. Given the range of topics addressed in epidemiologic research, there is likely to be a plurality of causal mechanisms. Researchers should not assume that there is one correct or optimal framework for causality that accounts for causal relationships identified in epidemiologic research. As Cartwright [23] observed, "Causation... is a highly varied thing. What causes should be expected to do and how they do it–really, what causes are–can vary from one kind of system of causal relations to another." Causation is not a single concept and many competing theories of causality have been proposed [23-26]. If we also accept that there are different kinds of causation with different features, then we must consider which methods are appropriate for which kinds of causation [23].

Overviews of quantitative models for identifying causal associations (such as the one included earlier in this volume) indicate that there are several approaches that are likely to be of use for epidemiologic research including structural equations modeling and the potential-outcomes model or counterfactual model. As noted previously, both probabilistic and deterministic models of disease causation can be linked to sufficient-component models of disease causation. In fields as diverse as philosophy of science and epidemiology, writers have conceptualized causality using deterministic models, quasi-deterministic models, and probabilistic models. Although there has been debate over whether a probabilistic model is the best way to conceptualize causation or whether causation should be viewed as deterministic [27-29], these contrasting viewpoints can be reconciled if one accepts that causation is a highly varied thing. As Cartwright [23] observed, what causes should be expected to do and how they do it is likely to vary from one kind of system of causal relations to another. Thus, causation is not one monolithic concept [23]. In epidemiology, both probabilistic and deterministic models of causation are likely to have something to offer for thinking about the nature of causality.

In epidemiology, a probabilistic model of causation holds that a cause increases the probability that a disease or other adverse health condition will occur. Under this model, the occurrence of a disease in an individual may be a matter of chance, i.e., it is a stochastic or indeterministic process [29]. Under a probabilistic model of causation, a cause may be neither necessary nor sufficient for the disease to occur.

In contrast, a deterministic model holds that diseases have causes and if these causes are present at certain points of time or time periods then diseases will follow. Both probabilistic and deterministic models of disease causation can be linked to sufficient-component models of disease causation. Sufficient-component models of disease causation are especially suitable for understanding the complex causation of many chronic diseases which often have multifactorial etiologies [26, 30].

SUMMARY AND CONCLUSIONS

In summary, emerging paradigms in epidemiologic research that take into account different levels of organization can help to strengthen causal inference in observational research. However, several impediments remain to be addressed before the full potential of such multilevel studies can be realized. These impediments include the need for further refinement of quantitative models for causal inference that are suitable for emerging research paradigms. Optimal approaches to causal inference are not necessarily identical across epidemiology subdisciplines and researchers should not assume that there is one correct or optimal theory of causality that accounts for causal relationships identified in epidemiologic research. Additional theoretical and methodological work is needed to help ensure that the causality of associations identified in epidemiologic research is adequately assessed.

REFERENCES

[1]   Susser M. Causal Thinking in the Health Sciences: Concepts and Strategies of Epidemiology. New York: Oxford University Press, 1973.

[2]   Terris M. The changing relationships of epidemiology and society. The Robert Cruikshank Lecture. J Public Health Policy 1985;6:15-36.

[3]   Ioannidis JP, Boffetta P, Little J, *et al.* Assessment of cumulative evidence on genetic associations: interim guidelines. Int J Epidemiol 2008;37:120-32.

[4]   Rubin DB. Estimating causal effects of treatments in randomized and nonrandomized studies. J Educ Psychol 1974;66:688-701.

[5]   Maldonado G, Greenland S. Estimating causal effects. Int J Epidemiol 2002;31:422-9.

[6]   Pearl J. Causality. New York: Springer, 2000.

[7]   Robins J, Greenland S. The probability of causation under a stochastic model for individual risk. Biometrics 1989;45:1125-38.

[8]   Little RJ, Rubin DB. Causal effects in clinical and epidemiological studies via potential outcomes: concepts and analytical approaches. Annu Rev Public Health 2000;21:121-45.

[9]   Greenland S. Causal analysis in the health sciences. J Am Stat Assoc 2000;95:286-9.

[10]   McMichael AJ. Prisoners of the proximate: loosening the constraints on epidemiology in an age of change. Am J Epidemiol 1999;149:887-97.

[11]   Diez Roux AV. Next steps in understanding the multilevel determinants of health. J Epidemiol Commun Health 2008;62:957-9.

[12]   Coughlin SS. Multilevel analysis in health services research (editorial). Open Health Serv Policy J 2009;2:42-44.

[13]   Leischow SJ, Milstein B. Systems thinking and modeling for public health practice. Am J Public Health 2006;96:403-5

[14]   Susser M, Susser E. Choosing a future for epidemiology: II. From black box to Chinese Boxes and eco-epidemiology. Am J Public Health 1996;86:674-7.

[15]   Krieger N. Epidemiology and the web of causation: has anyone seen the spider? Soc Sci Med 1994;39:887-903.

[16]   Glass TA, McAttee MJ. Behavioral science at the crossroads in public health: extending horizons, envisioning the future. Soc Sci Med 2006;62:1650-71.

[17]   Hafeman DM, Schwartz S. Opening the black box: a motivation for the assessment of mediation. Int J Epidemiol 2009:38:838-45.

[18]   Greenland S, Brumback B. An overview of relations among causal modeling methods. Int J Epidemiol 2002;31:1030-7.

[19]   Oakes JM. The (mis)estimation of neighborhood effects: causal inference for a practicable social epidemiology. Social Sci Med 2004;58:1929-52.

[20]   Factor-Litvak P, Sher A. Coming out of the box. Am J Epidemiol 2009;169:1179-81.

[21]   Hafeman DM, Schwartz S. Opening the black box: a motivation for the assessment of mediation. Int J Epidemiol 2009:38:838-45.

[22]   Hernan MA, Cole SR. Causal diagrams and measurement bias. Am J Epidemiol 2009;170:959-62.

[23]   Cartwright N. Hunting Causes and Using Them. Approaches in Philosophy and Economics. New York: Cambridge University Press, 2007.

[24]   Suppes P. A Probabilistic Theory of Causality. Amsterdam: North-Holland

Publishing Company, 1970.

[25]   Eells E. Probabilistic Causality. Cambridge, UK: Cambridge University Press, 1991.

[26]   Mackie J. The Cement of the Universe. Oxford: Clarendon Press, 1974.

[27]   Olsen J. What characterizes a useful concept of causation in epidemiology? J Epidemiol Commun Health 2003;57:86-88.

[28]   Karhausen LR. Causation: the elusive grail of epidemiology. Med Health Care Philos 2000;3:59-67.

[29]   Parascandola M, Weed DL. Causation in epidemiology. J Epidemiol Commun Health 2001;55:905-12.

[30]   Rothman KM. Causal inference in epidemiology. In: Modern Epidemiology. Boston: Little, Brown and Company, 1986.

SUBJECT INDEX

www.ingramcontent.com/pod-product-compliance
Lightning Source LLC
Chambersburg PA
CBHW041723210326
41598CB00007B/760